The Honey Revolution Series

Part 3

–

Feed Your Brain First

Feed Your Brain First

Part 3 - The Honey Revolution Series

Ronald E Fessenden, MD, MPH

TGBTGBooks.com, LLC
Colorado Springs, CO
2013

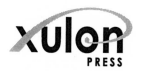

Table of Contents

Note to the Reader

Honey is a healthful food to be sure, but it cannot reverse what months and years of dietary indiscretions and lifestyle choices have caused. Regular honey consumption, especially at bedtime, will result in changes in sleep patterns and reduce nighttime metabolic stress almost immediately for most individuals. However, many disease processes as well as their ultimate prognoses may not be reversible or subject to midcourse correction.

The information provided in this book is not intended to be a substitute for the advice and counsel of your personal physician. Suggestions regarding the use of honey are recommendations, not prescriptions or medical guidelines for self-treatment and should not be substituted for any treatment recommendations prescribed by your physician. While the recommendations are appropriate and risk-free for most people, each individual may have differing requirements and/or responses to dietary recommendations based on one's complete medical profile.

The reader should also note that reductions in risks for any disease or condition are determined across large populations and do not necessarily apply to each individual within that population.

Finally, throughout the pages of this book, short "Stories" of real people appear. The metabolic profiles are based on individuals, but the names have been changed. Some profiles are composites representative of several individuals, all sharing the same or similar facts.

Acknowledgments

This is a book that would never have been written without the contributions of Mike McInnes, MRPS, a retired pharmacist from Edinburgh, Scotland. Mike's brilliance first came to my attention when I was handed a copy of *The Hibernation Diet* several years ago. The moment was accompanied by a bit of irony and a lot of skepticism. Most folks (including physicians) know that people don't hibernate. So why that title? And why should I be interested in another faddish diet plan?

Discovery of the answers to those questions was the first step in what resulted in the publication of three books. The first was the U.S. edition of *The Hibernation Diet,* for which I was privileged to write the Foreword and edit several additional pages left out of the original book by the publisher. The other two books were co-authored by Mike and myself (*The Honey Revolution - Restoring the Health of Future Generations*[1] and *The Honey Revolution - Abridged*[1]). This experience forever changed my understanding of human nutrition (if I ever had an understanding) and contributed to my knowledge of human physiology (again, a limited knowledge to be sure).

Mike's critical yet practical insights into the way our bodies metabolize and store carbohydrates underscored facts that have escaped medical scrutiny for decades. Combined with his exhaustive literature research over the past 15 years or so, these insights have allowed Mike to articulate a fueling strategy focused on honey and liver glycogen storage that will revolutionize medical practice once these facts make their way into clinical practice.

I first heard Mike present his theories at the First International Symposium on Honey and Health in Sacramento in January of 2008. Some of these, such as the fact that honey contains "anti-sugar signaling devices" (we know these now as factors that regulate "hepatic insulin signaling substance") that affect the way honey is differentiated, digested, and stored in the body quite differently than sucrose and high fructose corn syrup (HFCS), are already being evidenced in medical research of the past two to three years. As folks realize that proper nutrition based on producing and maintaining liver glycogen stores that fuel the brain are more important than blood sugar measurements or diets based on the Glycemic Index, more of his theories will be validated.

Portions of several chapters of this book were submitted by Mike in preliminary draft and much of the information contained throughout the book comes from our previous publications based on his literature research. For all of that and his friendship, I am grateful.

One other individual deserves special acknowledgement for his contributions to the advancement of the information contained in this book and in previous works by the author. Jerry Brown is a commercial beekeeper from North Central Kansas who invited me to join him in his company over six years ago. He was

responsible for first introducing me to Mike McInnes. Jerry has believed for some time that honey is more than just a sweetener and that the message of honey's healthful benefits needs to be front and center in promoting honey sales across the U.S. and beyond. With much gratitude, and after many years of compiling data and writing, I simply agree.

Many sincere thanks go to several other individuals who read and edited the manuscript, made comments, and emptied pens of red ink in the process. These include my lovely wife, Joyce, Paul Northen, who not only is a great editor but also a wonderful first tenor in Big Blue (the sanctuary choir of First Presbyterian Church of Colorado Springs) and his wife Pam, whose merciless, yet necessary editing, helped make this book what it is.

Finally, I want to acknowledge the Creator of all good things, the Lord of my life and the One in whom we all can have life and hope and joy - Jesus Christ. If there be any wisdom in this book, may God get the glory.

Foreword

*T*here are as many ways to read a book, as there are readers. In the case of this work, a suggestion or two may be in order.

Not everyone, I am told, appreciates detail. Nor is everyone impressed with fifty-cent words and phrases. While it is not my intent to include excessive detail or attempt to impress the reader with medical jargon, I must confess that a bit of my education and medical practice creeps into my writing now and then. And try as she might, my wife has not been successful in ridding this book of what may be viewed as incomprehensible and perhaps excessively didactic informational overflow.

For these and other reasons, I have begun each chapter with a section called Fast Track. If one considers only these sections, this book may be read in a little under three minutes, without missing any salient points.

For those with a more robust intellectual curiosity, or those who simply look to reading as a way of inducing a deep anesthetic state, the rest of the chapters are included. No specific regard has been given to expanding the total word count. If the stream of consciousness recital, however, becomes uninteresting, the reader is invited to revert to the Fast Track sections.

There have been many biblically based diet plans written and published over the years. *Feed Your Brain First* is not one of them. That is, this diet plan is not based on any specific dietary laws given to us in the Old Testament, nor does it draw from nutritional guidelines inferred from the Scriptures.

There is one biblical curiosity, however, that is explained, in part, in this book. Twenty seven times the phrase "milk and honey" is found in the Old Testament scriptures. Casual reading would seem to indicate that this reference simply underscores God's abundant nutritional provision for the early nomadic tribes of Israel. Milk was as available as the proximity of herds of cattle and goats that traveled with them. Honey was found in the rocks and crags of nearby hills, available for the taking, as needed, for food.

Yet, there is another truth about "milk and honey" that can be noted. Both contain natural sugars that fuel the brain. As we will see throughout this book, both fructose and glucose (the primary sugars found in honey) and lactose (the primary sugar found in milk which becomes galactose and glucose during digestion), work in similar ways to store glycogen (glucose) in the liver[2] — the primary fuel reserve for the brain. This is no small or hidden coincidence.

One additional note: the editorial style used throughout this book varies from first person - referencing the author — to a more generic third person - indicating no particular collection of folks. Perhaps this is because in the last 40 years of experience as a physician, I have come to understand that "nothing is new under the sun." Somewhere, someone has said something similar or at least thought it. The editorial "we" is simply a humble recognition that nothing new is being presented by one author alone, but rather represents the collective wisdom of many.

Ronald E Fessenden, MD, MPH

Introduction

*G*ood carbs, bad carbs . . . what's the difference? Are some carbs better for you? The diet industry and even some in the scientific community would have you believe so.

The glycemic index (GI) is called by some a "scientifically proven" index that seemingly justifies the consumption of certain carbohydrate intake over others. In other words, some carbs may be better for you than others simply by the time it takes for them to get broken down into glucose in the body. Are they?

This book takes you beyond the GI. It will inform you about a more important index of carbohydrate metabolism and show you how to make it work for you. It all starts with the brain.

The human brain exists in a state of "tension" every minute of the 24-hour cycle. It stands on constant alert with respect to the provision of its primary energy supply – glucose. The lack of a significant glucose storage facility in the brain makes this the most important consideration facing the brain at all times. A constant supply of glucose delivered to the brain by the circulating blood is critical.

During periods between meals, when no new energy is being ingested, the brain relies on two vital sources of glucose: blood glucose, the small amount of glucose constantly circulating in the blood; and liver glycogen, glucose stored in the liver. As blood glucose is delivered to and taken up by the brain and other peripheral tissues, the amount of glucose in the blood tends to fall (which if not corrected will result in a condition known as hypoglycemia or low blood sugar). This condition, if persistent, would quickly threaten brain function and eventually brain survival. The liver glycogen reserve, however, is able to release glucose into the circulation so that blood glucose concentration is maintained, usually within a very narrow range.[3]

As the blood glucose level falls, the brain triggers the release of adrenaline, a hormone from the adrenal glands. Adrenaline activates an enzyme in the liver[4] that cleaves the starchy glycogen globule into single glucose units so that these may be released into circulation.

There is one other major glycogen storage area in the human body that deserves mention. This reserve contains more than ten times the amount of glycogen as the liver. This is the primary store considered by athletes, glucose stored in muscle cells as glycogen. Muscle cells, however, lack the enzyme contained in liver cells and therefore are unable to release glucose back into the blood for use by the brain or any other organ when blood glucose concentration falls. Muscle glycogen is reserved exclusively for use within muscle cells and is used to power contracting muscles only during exercise.

In the period during and after a meal that includes a large percentage of carbohydrates, blood glucose concentration rises rapidly. Insulin is released from the beta cells of the pancreas gland to drive glucose into peripheral tissues so that glucose homeostasis (stability) is maintained. High blood glucose (hyperglycemia) is a very dangerous condition, and a quick insulin response is vital in this situation. In healthy metabolism, this rapid insulin release prompts a quick return of blood sugar (blood glucose concentration) to normal levels.

The glycemic index (GI) was created to provide a measure of how different carbohydrate foods affect this response. In other words, the GI indicates how rapidly carbohydrates get into the blood and elevate the blood sugar. The higher the GI, the more rapidly glucose from carbohydrate ingestion raises the blood glucose level.

Unfortunately, the blood glucose concentration (whether low, normal or high) after the ingestion of these foods provides us with no indication of the quantity of liver glycogen that may be available to fuel the brain in the period between meals or during the nighttime. This is the measure or index that is of vital interest to the brain. If the liver glycogen store is low, the ability of the liver to replenish falling blood glucose levels and thereby maintain glucose supply to the brain is immediately compromised.

The Brain Fuel Status Indicator

Our bodies do have a brain fuel status indicator that few know about. It serves a purpose similar to the "low fuel" light on our car's instrument panel. This metabolic "warning light" alerts the brain to an impending fuel shortage. One would think that this important critical index of brain energy status would be understood and emphasized in every physician's office, every patient care setting, on a routine basis. Surprisingly, such is not the case!

The fact that the liver and brain have such an early warning signal should surprise no one. The brain has no energy store of its own and would survive for only a few seconds if its outside fuel supply were cut off. The amount of glucose contained in the blood at any one time is only about five grams, enough to provide energy for a few minutes of brain function. Together, the amount of glucose in the blood and small the amount of glucose in the glial cells that transport fuel to the brain represent only a transient supply of fuel. Therefore, any measure that indicates the rate that glucose may be available to the blood, such as the GI, is only of passing and limited value as far as the brain is concerned.

This brain fuel status indicator is known as insulin-like growth factor-binding protein-1[5] (IGFBP-1). In this book it will be referred to as the *brain fuel indicator* or *BFI*. The BFI is an easily measured "index" of liver glycogen availability and inversely indicates the status of fuel available for the brain at any given moment. This indicator introduces a new dynamic for understanding glycemic (blood sugar) control. It opens a new paradigm for monitoring, indexing, and correcting conditions and diseases of impaired energy metabolism and consequently all the major degenerative metabolic diseases that are draining resources in our increasingly beleaguered health care systems.

The BFI is a much improved "glycemic index" representing a major step forward in dietary and nutritional recommendations as well as in developing new strategies for combating all the diseases and conditions of the metabolic syndrome. I am increasingly confident that the use of the BFI in routine clinical medicine will yield positive results in opposing the national and international public health challenges that afflict not only adult, elderly, and relatively inactive populations, but also increasingly affect an ever-widening spectrum of the whole population, including children, and more surprisingly even reaching sections of the athletic community.

The challenge for today in using the BFI as an index is not simple or routine. Most physicians would not know that the BFI (the actual level of IGFBP-1 measured by a simple blood test) is inversely proportional to the amount of glycogen contained in the liver. Furthermore, it is not currently "routine" to test for IGFBP-1 in clinical medicine.

The good news is that it is not necessary to actually analyze blood for IGFBP-1 to know what is happening to the liver glycogen reserve. So, you might ask, what is the purpose of having an index if you don't need to know what it is?

Fortunately, our understanding of glucose metabolism and storage allows us to know a lot about the liver glycogen reserve and how to ensure that the tank is full without having to measure it. That is what this book is all about.

Chapter 1

Fast Track
• Glucose is the primary fuel that the brain utilizes for its energy needs.
• The brain has no way to store glucose and must depend on the circulating blood to deliver glucose to it at all times.
• The brain regulates its own energy supply and demand to ensure production of new glucose when blood sugar levels are low.
• The process used by the brain to initiate the production of new glucose involves the release of adrenalin and cortisol, a process referred to in this book as *metabolic stress*.
• *Metabolic stress*, a brain-protective mechanism, is caused by brain hunger.
• The glycemic index (GI), based on blood sugar, is extremely transient and provides no advance notice to the brain of its depleted energy supply.

> - There is an indicator of the brain's fuel supply, referred to as the brain fuel indicator (BFI).
> - Optimization of the BFI reduces metabolic stress.

Fuel for a Hungry Brain

*T*he human brain depends on glucose, the most essential carbohydrate in human metabolism. That is, each and every brain cell (neuron) relies almost exclusively on a continuous and uninterrupted supply of glucose for energy and life. Only in very exceptional metabolic circumstances is the brain able to metabolize other fuels (namely lactate and ketones) and only then when glucose is in short supply. All other cells and tissues within the human body are not so metabolically challenged; that is to say, they may metabolize (use for energy) carbohydrates, fats and proteins, but not the brain.

Part of the reason for the brain's selectivity in fuel is that the human brain is separated or protected from the general circulation by what is called the blood-brain barrier. This highly selective partition is structured to allow only certain molecules to pass over from the blood plasma into the brain's circulation. For example, fats or fatty acids are prevented from crossing the blood-brain barrier and are therefore not available for direct energy provision for the brain. Likewise, proteins and their precursors, amino acids, are subject to selective filtering by this barrier. Those amino acids that can cross over are utilized, not for energy, but for other metabolic requirements. Glucose crosses this barrier quite easily and for this reason is the brain's primary source of fuel.

In addition to this predilection for glucose, the brain's demand for fuel and energy exceeds that of all other organs and tissues in the human body by a mighty factor of 20. This distinction qualifies the human brain as the highest energy consuming tissue yet discovered.

The Empty Brain

"The brain has no significant energy storage facility itself, and must . . . compete with all other organs and tissues for a sustained energy supply."

In spite of its colossal energy demand, the human brain manifests a surprising and unique metabolic distinction. The brain has no significant energy storage facility itself and must therefore, at all times, compete with all other organs and tissues for a sustained energy supply to maintain its metabolic life. The brain carries only a 30-second fuel reserve in the star-shaped glial cells of the brain-brain barrier.[6] Actually, if the blood glucose supply to the brain was somehow abruptly cut off, the brain's small glycogen reserve could theoretically last for several minutes. However, within 30 seconds, brain cells would begin to die off. Therefore, the 30-second window of survival remains a valid working model for the living human brain.

Fortunately the brain is blessed with a unique capacity to regulate energy supply and demand within the human body. It does so by assuming absolute command and control over all energy intake and storage, including the appetite that drives food intake and the storage and selection of fuels, placing its own requirements as the first and overriding priority.

This competition and regulation over which the brain exercises control extends to the actual

"cannibalization" of other peripheral tissues, if necessary, when glucose is in short supply. This means that
the brain orchestrates a condition in which tissues are
degraded and converted into new glucose (gluconeogenesis).[7] Fats are not used to make glucose under any
conditions. The primary source of substances used by
the body to make this new glucose is protein derived
from muscle tissue.

The regulatory system involved with activating
this process is responsible for the physiology of *metabolic stress.*[8] When this system is activated, hormones
(cortisol and adrenalin) are released from the adrenal
glands that deplete the liver glycogen store of any
stored glucose and initiate the process of converting
protein from the muscles into new glucose for the brain.

Cerebral Hunger - the Driver of Metabolic Stress

*"Metabolic stress is exclusively driven by brain
hunger."*

It is important to underscore this relationship
between the brain's energy demand and a condition
described throughout this book as *metabolic stress.*
Other forms of stress discussed at length in popular and
scientific texts refer to environmental and psychosocial
stress. These types of stress activate the same reactive
physiology but not to the degree that internal metabolic stress does. The brain initiates internal metabolic
stress when it senses that its fuel supply is running low
(brain hunger).

The key to understanding stress physiology is in
knowing that this is the mechanism utilized by the brain
to make glucose for its own energy needs whenever

glucose is in short supply. In typical medical practice today, the most immediate measure or index for this energy availability is the blood glucose concentration or blood sugar, as it is known in lay terms. But as we shall see, this is not a very reliable indicator of brain fuel reserve.

"The popular Glycemic Index (GI) is not 'proven science.'"

Throughout the 1900s, diabetes research has deemed the blood glucose measure a kind of "Holy Grail" and seemingly elevated its status to one of pseudo-academic importance. This observation is confirmed by noting the widespread use of the glucose tolerance test (GTT) during the mid to later part of the 20th century. The GTT and the fasting blood glucose concentration were commonly used as the major indicators of metabolic health. This in turn led to the development of the Glycemic Index (GI). The GI (the relative effect of various carbohydrate foods on blood glucose concentration) took on somewhat of a mythic status in that it became the theoretical basis for a number of weight control diets, and was/is promoted enthusiastically by various dietary gurus.

This approach could be described as interesting as it does provide useful information on various foods, but it is not a major scientific breakthrough in any sense, nor should it be rightly touted as "proven science."

More recently, the GI has come under increasing scrutiny, in particular from the perspective of the basis for its definition. The GI is based on blood glucose, a profoundly transient or short-term measure. In economic terms, the GI may be illustrated by comparing the difference between a current bank account and a savings account. If a person's current account is low or even in negative balance, but the savings account from which it may be replenished is in good order, the prognosis remains good. If however, the savings account is low or empty there is most certainly a problem as the current bank account nears depletion. As spending continues, new sources of funding will have to be found to replenish reserves.

The "brain fuel indicator" (BFI) is more relevant than the glycemic index (GI).

The liver glycogen store, the only reserve that may release glucose for cerebral energy in the periods between meals, is the glycemic equivalent of the savings account, at least from the perspective of the human brain. The liver glycogen store is very small, averaging around 75 to 80 grams. Yet this small store provides enough fuel reserve for the brain for up to eight hours without being replenished. Therefore, a more significant index for the human brain in terms of its energy supply and survival is what we refer to as the liver glycogen index or the *brain fuel indicator* (BFI) rather than the glycemic index (GI).

In *Feed Your Brain First*, we will demonstrate why the failure of the various health professions to take this critical measure into account has resulted in a marked increase in the prevalence of the diseases of metabolic impairment, including heart disease, diabetes, obesity and other neuro-degenerative conditions. Furthermore, we will show how this vital index can be optimized by selective fuel replenishment, resulting in the provision of cerebral energy at critical times, thus resulting in the reduction of metabolic stress and therefore a reduced risk for all the metabolic diseases. And finally, we will give you practical ways to stock this vital storehouse with glucose through recipes and menus that will help prevent or eliminate metabolic stress altogether.

Tom's Story

*A*t age 22, Tom was a picture of fitness and health: 74 inches tall, 180 pounds wet, sculpted abs and upper torso, powerful legs and muscular arms. He had completed college, married and in time entered the workforce as an investment broker, becoming chained to a desk with a computer terminal for hours each day for weeks on end that extended into years and then into decades. In his late 20s, he had become a runner, putting in 20 to 30 miles a week on the track or treadmill. He had even completed a couple of marathons.

Since then, he had given up exercise in exchange for many of life's more sedentary and supine pleasures.

Time Changes Things

Now at age 55, time and lifestyle had taken a toll. Tom weighed in at 270 pounds; his body still sculpted but in a more "settled" and rounded way. His health was measured by numbers, not miles on the track – numbers like 260 (cholesterol) and 7.6 (HbA1c or glycohemoglobin) and 150/96 (blood pressure).

In addition to the obvious changes in Tom's appearance, something more sinister was taking place within

Tom's body, something that Tom could not appreciate, except on what were becoming increasingly more frequent occasions.

Sleep patterns were changing and his wife complained about an increase in snoring. Tolerance for mild to moderate exercise was decreasing. Midday fatigue and excessive sleepiness were beginning to affect work. He was always hungry, or so it seemed, consuming snacks and soft drinks throughout the day. Mornings were miserable as he awakened feeling shaky, fatigued and often nauseous, able only to gulp down a cup of coffee before heading out the door to work.

Tom's story is a classic illustration of life in the 21st century for thousands, even millions of folks. Tom's doctor diagnosed Type 2 diabetes, hyperlipidemia (elevated cholesterol and triglycerides) and hypertension (high blood pressure), politely leaving out obesity, and prescribed several pills to treat his "diseases" and control his numbers. [This approach characterizes much of modern medicine. "Treat the numbers" rather than the cause.]

The truth is that Tom was experiencing *chronic partial brain starvation* coupled with *chronic partial sleep loss* and *endogenous metabolic stress*. In fact, he had been experiencing these relatively unknown conditions for years. Unfortunately for Tom, the "treatment" was just as likely to be unknown as the diagnoses. In subsequent pages, we will break down these unfamiliar terms and show you why they are more accurate "diagnoses" than the ones Tom's doctor used, but for now let's get back to Tom's story.

To unravel the genesis of Tom's progressively deteriorating health, role back the clock and take another picture of Tom – a word picture that looks at what's taking place on the inside rather than the exterior.

This is a picture that you won't find described in any medical chart or textbook, yet nevertheless, one that is just as important, perhaps more important than if Tom's doctor had written it.

An Inside Look

"The liver is at the heart of Tom's progressively poor health."

The picture that you are about to have revealed is really quite simple. It focuses on one organ – the liver – and its role in providing fuel for the brain. Admittedly, the liver is not a very sexy organ. It is seldom publically portrayed in any disease scenario except the conditions caused by alcohol, infectious agents or cancer. No one inquires about the liver in casual conversations like they might about the heart or stomach or other more visible body parts. Yet the liver is at the heart of Tom's progressively poor health.

Here's why. You see, Tom was genetically predisposed to be a 180-pound male. His body parts, including his internal organs, were perfectly proportioned to support and sustain a man at that weight. At maturity, his *liver* weighed approximately 1.6 kg (3.5 pounds) and could manufacture and store about 80 to 90 grams of glycogen at any given time, enough to sustain his brain, kidneys and red blood cells through eight hours or so of sleep or one hour of intense physical exercise.

At age 55, Tom's metabolic demands were increased by at least one-third over those at age 22, perhaps by as much as 50%. His resting heart rate was faster. His blood pressure was up as his heart had to pump blood through more than 9,000 miles of additional blood vessels now circulating blood through the additional 90 pounds of fat.

Keeping Up with Demand Only Makes Things Worse

Part of the fuel for this increased demand could be made up for by increased consumption. For several years, Tom tried to keep pace; but the more he consumed, the more demand he placed on his metabolic requirements and the more glucose intolerant he became. Furthermore, the more carbohydrates Tom consumed, the greater was his demand for insulin production, and the less effective his insulin became in partitioning glucose into the cells (his body was becoming "insulin resistant").

In addition, Tom's fat stores were themselves colossal consumers of glucose, requiring increased amounts of energy just to maintain the hugely increased storage capacity. Tom's liver glycogen store was being depleted at an excessive rate, just to maintain peripheral fat deposits!

The Starving Brain Is a Greedy Brain

Instead of having enough glycogen in his liver for eight hours of sleep, Tom's brain fuel reserve tank was running on low. Compounded by poor eating habits, and the failure to restock his liver before bedtime with glycogen (we'll tell you how to do that in another chapter), Tom was experiencing *partial nocturnal brain starvation* night after night. Another way to say this is that Tom's brain was "out of gas." Tom's brain reacted to this energy deficit by initiating a protective mechanism called *metabolic stress*. That means that his brain triggered the release of the adrenal hormones, adrenalin and cortisol, to ensure adequate fuel for the brain during a time when no food was being ingested. Metabolic stress awakened Tom early in the morning and resulted in poor quality and interrupted sleep or *chronic partial sleep loss.* (Adrenalin is not a sleeping aid.)

Excess cortisol released night after night, as in Tom's case, had a serious negative impact on his glucose metabolism rendering the insulin that his body did produce less effective over time. Eventually, this resulted in glucose intolerance, insulin resistance and Type 2 diabetes.

Tom's excessive consumption of calories over the years had resulted in a condition we call *partial brain starvation.* This resulted in even more demands for energy, more consumption of food, more metabolic stress, poor quality sleep, and increased risk for the dreaded diseases of aging including memory impairments and Alzheimer's disease. Tom had entered the downward spiral of life experienced prematurely by so many in midlife.

When the Liver Is the "Heart" of the Problem

Earlier, we said that the liver was at the heart of Tom's problem. Let's connect a few more dots. As Tom reached physical maturity, his liver size and capacity to store glycogen topped out at about 80 to 90 grams. At age 55, his liver glycogen storage capacity was still only 80 to 90 grams, possibly a bit less as dietary abuses over the years, such as the excessive consumption of high fructose corn syrup (HFCS), would have contributed to a fatty liver.[9] Alcohol use may have also decreased the ability of his liver to process and store glucose.

Liver glycogen is the one critical fuel reserve for the brain, red blood cells and the kidneys. Liver glycogen also serves as fuel reserve for every other cell in the body when blood sugar is low. At rest, a normal liver can release up to ten grams of glucose per hour to the rest of the body to help meet its metabolic needs.

During the midlife years and later, Tom's need for liver glycogen was increased above the norm. Instead of ten grams per hour at rest, Tom's body demanded significantly more glycogen per hour to sustain his brain, red blood cells and kidneys, but also the increasing peripheral mass of tissue he had accumulated over the years.

When Tom retired for bed after the late evening TV news, his liver glycogen store was already partially depleted. His last meal, consumed about 6:00 PM, may have added some to the glycogen store, but by bedtime, Tom may have had only 30 to 40 grams of liver glycogen remaining, enough for only three to four hours of brain fuel during sleep. By 2:30 AM his liver was signaling his brain that a fuel crisis was nearing. His brain reacted in the normal way to secure a new food supply by waking Tom up with an adrenalin and cortisol release, designed to produce new glucose from his body's protein.

Starving in the Land of Plenty

Tom's system was flush with fuel all the time. He ate excessively and frequently. His blood sugar levels were consistently high, compatible with his food intake. His fat stores were abundant and constantly being renewed and replenished. He lived with an abundance of stored energy. *The sad irony was that Tom's brain was increasingly and repeatedly being starved*. Medication for his diabetes, hyperlipidemia and hypertension did nothing to correct his underlying problem. His treatment was directed at reducing his "numbers" rather than correcting the cause.

His brain was constantly competing for fuel with his increasing body mass and the result was repeated nighttime metabolic stress. His liver was unable to create and store glycogen because of metabolic stress and therefore unable to stock sufficient fuel reserve for the brain for the night or even for daytime use.

Every Man's (and Every Woman's) Story

"Tom's story is a medical metaphor for what is experienced by millions of Americans."

Tom's story is not unique. The specific numbers and the progression of the pathology may vary somewhat from person to person, male to female, but generally, Tom is a medical metaphor for millions of Americans diagnosed with adult onset diabetes (Type 2 diabetes), insulin resistance, obesity, hypertension, hyperlipidemia, cardiovascular disease, osteoporosis, and even Alzheimer's disease.

Not everyone will share Tom's experience. There are many factors that influence the manifestation of disease and the intensity or severity of symptoms. Certainly genetics play an important role, as do diet, lifestyle, environmental exposure and many other factors.

Yet the truth is that many of the diseases and conditions afflicting 21st century folks are variations of that experienced by Tom. They all have their origins in what physicians have referred to since the 1990s as *the metabolic syndrome*. At the center of all of these diseases and conditions are three common threads: *chronic partial nocturnal (brain) starvation, chronic partial sleep loss* and *chronic intermittent metabolic stress.*[10]

The way these threads intertwine and manifest themselves in people may vary across a wide range of outcomes, yet all share the same causal elements. Not everyone who is overweight gets diabetes. Not every one who is skinny has normal blood glucose metabolism. Some develop osteoporosis. Some have thyroid deficiency. Others are depressed. Many are destined to have an early onset of Alzheimer's disease or Parkinsonism or other forms of neuro-degenerative diseases, some even at an early age. Some get cancer or coronary artery disease. Many have hypertension or become handicapped from strokes. Others just sleep poorly every night.

The interventions and therapies that are served up by contemporary medicine to combat these diseases and conditions are multiple and varied, and (do we have to state the obvious?), expensive! The direct and indirect costs for diabetes alone are approaching $200 billion a year just in the United States.

Wouldn't it be better to just prevent these things from occurring in the first place? What a preposterous idea you may think. Just give me a pill! But pills treat the numbers and do little to change underlying causes of disease. If the truth be known and given wide acceptance in medicine, all of the diseases and conditions mentioned above may be simply prevented. In many cases, the progression of symptoms may easily be reversed or arrested.

Chapter 2

Fast Track

- The most important consideration in nutrition and diet is fueling the brain.
- Blood sugar readings tell us little or nothing about the status of the brain's fuel reserve.
- Nutritional advice (especially relating to carbohydrates) believed to be true during the past four decades has produced more obesity, diabetes, and neuro-degenerative diseases than during any other time in the history of our nation.
- All carbohydrates are sugars. Glucose is the *king* of carbohydrates.
- The average American gets more than ten times the amount of calories from sugars than recommended by major health organizations.
- While carbohydrates are not essential nutrients in humans, one carbohydrate (glucose) is essential for the brain.
- Excess carbohydrates are stored in the body as fat.

Fuel the brain first!

"Proper fueling of the brain is more important than blood sugar measurements or calories or carbohydrates or fats or anything else related to nutrition for that matter."

*L*et's get this right from the start! When discussing the types of foods we eat and the timing of when we eat them, the most important consideration is how best to fuel the brain. Nothing else should take top priority. Proper fueling of the brain is more important than blood sugar measurements or calories or carbohydrates or fats or anything else related to nutrition for that matter. Yet fueling the brain is seldom, if ever, mentioned in nutrition and dietary counseling, and we would wager that no one has ever heard their physicians mention lack of proper brain fuel as a cause for anything.

Failure to fuel the brain properly throughout the day and night is the number one cause for most of what ails us in today's culture. Since the 1990s, medicine has lumped these associated conditions and diseases together and given them the label of the "metabolic syndrome." These conditions and diseases include obesity, diabetes, hyperlipidemia, heart and blood pressure abnormalities, osteoporosis, hypothyroidism and several other challenges to health that we will describe later in Chapter 8. All of these are related to, associated with, or otherwise caused by the lack of proper and timely energy for a hungry brain. We will explain how this happens in subsequent chapters.

Already we can hear the protests. How in an age of overindulgence and excessive intake – the evidence is clear from people watching most everywhere – can the brain be hungry? It is so counterintuitive to state that brain starvation could possibly exist in an era of excess consumption, yet such is indeed the case. The way we eat, what we eat, and when we eat, are factors contributing to brain starvation, something that occurs on a daily basis for a majority of people. This book will show you why this is true and help you to know what to do about it.

Treating the Numbers

The advancements in medical science over the past couple of decades have produced a sense of false hope. Without question, therapeutic strategies mostly by way of pharmaceutical interventions can "treat the numbers." Drugs can lower your cholesterol (or even particular fractions of total cholesterol), control your blood sugar, stabilize your serotonin and glutamate (neurotransmitters) and increase your calcium without affecting the underlying cause of the metabolic stress that results in the conditions and diseases of the metabolic syndrome. In other words, medication may indeed treat your diseases and provide some sense of control, making our doctors and us happy while at the same time, the underlying causative condition (meta-bolic stress) rages on within our bodies.

"Blood sugar . . . is quite an irrelevant number . . . It tells us little or nothing about the status of the brain's primary fuel reserve."

In no area of medical practice is this dichotomy – the contrasting approach between treatment or control and the underlying cause of a condition – more focused than in the consideration of blood sugar or blood glucose. Over the past half a century blood sugar measurement has evolved into the *sine qua non* of human metabolism evaluation. Patients are informed that they are pre-diabetic or diabetic based on the value of this measurement and other associated lab values such as HbA1c.[11] Drug companies have made fortunes formulating medicines that can reduce the numbers and regulate blood sugar within a "normal range."

Yet if the whole truth were known, blood sugar, except in the extremes of both excessively high and low measurements, is quite an irrelevant number.[12] It is extremely transient and subject to strict regulation within the body. Blood sugar alone tells us little or nothing about the status of the brain's primary fuel reserve. In other words, the blood sugar measurement may be within a normal range while at the same instant, the brain's fuel supply is depleted placing the brain in imminent danger. The same may also be true when the blood glucose is elevated on a chronic basis. Such conditions exist for a large majority of folks every day and night for weeks at a time, without their knowledge and irrespective of blood sugar levels. The result is a metabolic condition that we have referred to above as metabolic stress.

To understand the reasons for this and what might be done about it, it is essential to establish a base of information regarding sugar or carbohydrate metabolism. In later chapters, we will describe the risks associated with chronic metabolic stress and detail the benefits of providing the brain with proper fuel throughout the day and how that may be accomplished.

Carbohydrates - What We Already Know

Why another discussion of carbohydrate metabolism and glucose regulation? Why does it matter? It matters because after more than a century of scientific study and clinical observation and practice, doctors and nutrition specialists still don't have it right.

"Nutritional advice that we believed to be true has produced more obesity, diabetes, and neuro-degenerative diseases than during any other time in the history of our nation."

The majority of us in the medical and scientific communities are badly uninformed, driven by pharmaceutical "solutions" and pressured by a results oriented "can't you just give me a pill, Doc?" society. The rest of us who depend on the experts to keep us healthy and provide us with up-to-date information are confused as we learn that nutritional advice that we believed to be true has produced more obesity, diabetes, and neuro-degenerative diseases than during any other time in the history of our nation.

What we do know is taking a very long time to make its way into practical conventional wisdom useful for everyday folks. There are many reasons for this. Oversight, ignorance, and marketing money from the processed foods industry – lots of it – are having a disastrous effect on our public health in epidemic proportions. Even our federal agencies that have all the data and should know better are complicit in not getting the correct information out! Professional organizations and associations that are controlled or strongly influenced by special interests - spell that *money* – focus on costly interventions well after the damage has been done, rather than on prevention.

Medical practice, generally speaking, prefers intervention and treatment over prevention. Yet for all the good it does, medicine is losing the war on obesity, diabetes, and the many other diseases and conditions directly caused by or associated with faulty or impaired glucose metabolism. The solutions are relatively simple. However, an almost universal blindness has succeeded in keeping what should have been apparent out of the mainstream of public health and medical practice.

It was 1901 and 1903 when the first significant observations were made linking glucose regulation to adrenal function.[13] Even before that in 1840, Dr. Claude Bernard described the first central nervous system response affecting blood glucose control.

These early studies and dozens that have followed in the succeeding decades have documented what should have been obvious. In spite of this seminal work carried out by Bernard in the mid 19th century and later by Dr. Noel Paton at the beginning of the 20th century and many more since then, *researchers have continued to ignore the liver and its key role in glucose storage, release and regulation.* This "liver blindness" is both a scientific and cultural phenomenon, inexplicable when one is confronted with a few simple facts.

Glucose - the King of Carbohydrates

Quite simply, carbohydrates are foods that are made up mostly of starch or sugar. We think of them primarily as plant based (that is they come from plants) with the one big exception being lactose, a sugar found in milk. Scientists think of carbohydrates synonymously with saccharides (or sugars) that exist either as singular molecules (monosaccharides such as glucose or fructose) or two or more molecules joined together (disaccharides such as sucrose or lactose, or oligosaccharides and polysaccharides such as starch or glycogen).

Underscore this fact: *carbohydrates are sugars*. And don't get confused by the "good carbs, bad carbs" debate. *Carbs are sugar. It's just that simple.*

Most of us know the foods that are high in carbohydrates. The list includes bread, potatoes, rice, whole grains, vegetables, pastas, cereals and most anything made from flour or corn or other grains. Carbohydrates are the most common source of energy in living organisms, and glucose is the *king* of carbohydrates. These foods are all high in starch. Starch is a polysaccharide made up of many molecules of glucose. Plants make starch as a way of storing sugar for energy for growth and reproduction. *Starch is glucose!*

Don't Be Deceived!

When you look on the nutrition facts label of any food product requiring such a label, starch is sometimes not listed but included as part of the total carbohydrates. Sometimes starch is listed separately from sugars, wrongly implying that starch is something other than sugar.

For example, if one looks at the nutrition facts for one large potato weighing about 300 grams, you will see that it contains 63 grams of carbohydrates and only four grams of sugar. Wouldn't you infer from this information that 59 grams of this potato were made up of something other than sugar? The truth is those 59 grams are composed of fiber (seven grams) and starch

(52 grams) which are sugars! This sleight of hand, whether intentional or not is quite deceptive to the food shopper who actually reads labels.

"The most important sugar in human metabolism is glucose, the saccharide that is found in the body as blood sugar."

It doesn't matter that we call them complex or simple carbs. Carbs are sugars. We'll get to the digestibility of starches and sugars and the Glycemic Index later, but for now, know that *carbohydrates are sugar!* The word sugar here refers to generic sugar, not specifically table sugar (or sucrose), but other sugars, simple or complex, single molecules or molecules linked together by a simple chemical bond that is easily broken during the process of digestion. The most important sugar in human metabolism is glucose, the saccharide that is found in the body as blood glucose.

Recommendations for the total percentage of dietary energy requirements that should be met from carbohydrates range from 45 to 75% depending on the organization making those recommendations.[14] Only 10% of our total daily energy requirements, expert nutritionists tell us, should come directly from sugars, meaning simple carbohydrates.[15] If you cannot differentiate starch or other carbohydrates from sugars on the nutrition label, how is it possible for you to know if you are meeting the recommended guidelines for sugar consumption? The fact is, it is not possible.

Furthermore, the average American obtains 60 to 80% of the necessary energy requirements (calories) from carbohydrates and more than 20 to 40% of those come from simple sugars. This excessive consumption traces its beginnings in part to the 1970s when high fructose corn syrup (HFCS) was first produced cheaply from cornstarch. Within a few years, HFCS became the sweetener of choice used by food manufactures and today represents 40% of the sweeteners used in foods and beverages. The most commonly used HFCS is composed of 55% fructose and 45% glucose. It is not really "high fructose" but rather a nearly equal ratio of fructose and glucose made from cornstarch.[16]

A conservative estimate of HFCS consumption today indicates that *the daily average for all Americans aged two and above is 330 grams or 1320 calories from HFCS alone.*[17] That's a whopping *0.73 pounds of HFCS a day* or 182 grams (0.4 pounds or 726 calories) from fructose and 148 grams (0.33 pounds or 594 calories) from glucose, two simple sugars whose combined total daily consumption should be limited to no more than 25 grams for women and 37 grams for men.[18] Stating this another way, *the average American female above the age of two consumes more than thirteen times the recommended amount of sugar from HFCS each day, and the average male nearly nine times the recommended amount.* Is there any question as to the cause of the national obesity epidemic? Common sense would indicate that there is a significant association.

Carbohydrate Consumption from HFCS

Average consumption per day =
330 grams (0.73 pounds)
Amount of simple sugars recommended
for adult males per day = **37 grams**
Amount or simple sugars recommended
for adult females per day = **25 grams**

Excess amount of simple sugars consumed per day
from HFCS = ~ 300 grams or nearly 2/3 pound for
every man, woman and child

Carbohydrates Are Nonessential

The fact that glucose is the *king* of carbohydrates stands in direct contradiction to the fact that *carbohydrates are not essential nutrients in humans.* The body can obtain all its energy requirements from proteins and fats! It's almost sacrilegious to repeat this statement, especially in our overindulgent carbohydrate-saturated society but *carbohydrates are not essential in the human diet.* The body can make all the glucose it requires for fuel out of proteins or amino acids. Other energy requirements can be met by fat. Sorry, all you vegans, vegetarians, and plant-based diet gurus out there, but your zealous pursuit of health and happiness through a highly selective vegetarian diet is based on nonessentials, at least as far as the logic of human metabolism is concerned.

One Carbohydrate (Glucose) Is Essential for the Brain

From the perspective of the brain, it may appear to be a significant irony to label carbohydrates as nonessential. After all, the brain and its individual cells (neurons) rely almost entirely on glucose for energy. It cannot burn fat except under limited and harsh conditions. Only in the second stage of starvation will the brain burn ketones ("fat bodies" or fat metabolites). Also, the brain will use certain amino acids from proteins for fuel, but only in small amounts. The brain uses glucose as its primary energy supply.

OK, to avoid any confusion, let's restate the facts.

1. All carbohydrates are sugars. Starches are carbohydrates. Starches are sugars.
2. Carbohydrates are **nonessential** for human metabolism and energy needs.
3. Glucose is a carbohydrate, a simple sugar.
4. Glucose *is essential* for brain fuel. In fact, it is the exclusive fuel selected by the brain for its energy needs.
5. The brain's requirement for glucose takes priority over all other metabolic considerations in the body.

So if the brain requires glucose, and we consume huge amounts of glucose (starches and other carbohydrates which get converted to glucose), that's good for the brain isn't it? What's the problem?

The answer lies in understanding how the body handles (or metabolizes) glucose. Excessive amounts of carbohydrates consumed daily are eventually converted to glucose in the digestive process. This amount of glucose simply overwhelms our systems, triggering a massive release of insulin which drives excess glucose into the cells where it is either used for energy or *stored as fat*. Once glucose enters muscle cells, whether it is used for energy or stored as fat, it is no longer available to the brain or for any other tissue or cell in the body. Another way to say this is that consumption of excessive amounts of carbohydrates leads to brain starvation.

Chapter 3

Fast Track

- Most carbohydrates are broken down or digested into glucose and stored as glycogen.
- The primary fuel reserve for the brain is the liver, where glucose is stored as glycogen.
- The average capacity of this brain fuel reserve is 75 grams.
- Focusing on the glycemic index (GI) in one's diet ignores the brain fuel supply.
- Consuming foods that contain an equal ratio of fructose and glucose (like honey, fruits and some vegetables) stock the brain fuel reserve.
- Too much fructose (more than 30 grams at any one time) may be harmful to your health.
- The 13 (often ignored) principles of fueling the brain, if followed, can prevent disease and improve health.

Carbohydrate Metabolism 101

Carbohydrate metabolism refers to the process by which carbs[19] or sugars are broken down or digested, formed or inter-converted into a different sugar, and stored as other carbohydrate forms within the body. It's not really very complicated.

Carbs are ingested. Enzymes in the saliva, stomach and GI tract break down the carbs (starch or sugars) into glucose. Glucose enters the blood stream and triggers a release of insulin from the pancreas. Insulin drives the glucose into the cells. Glucose is used by nearly every cell type in the body to create a substance called ATP.[20] The cells use ATP for the transfer of energy. Without ATP, cells lack energy and fail to function properly.

Many "complex" carbohydrates are not broken down in the upper GI tract and pass into the large intestine where bacteria and other enzymes work to digest them into simple sugars. These simple sugars can then be absorbed into the blood. Any undigested complex carbs (fibers and other complex carbs) are eliminated. The extra energy needed to complete this longer digestion process is actually quite insignificant. The end result is that most carbohydrates still end up as glucose.

When no glucose is available, either in the diet or from glucose stored as glycogen, the body must manufacture it out of amino acids that come from proteins. Glucose, whether directly ingested or digested from foods and absorbed from the GI tract or formed from amino acids, exists in the body either as circulating blood glucose or as glycogen, which is stored in the liver or muscle cells.

Carbohydrate Storage - Reservoir Management

Earlier, we stated that the brain's requirements for fuel take priority over all other metabolic considerations. The brain burns primarily glucose under normal circumstances. Given these facts, doesn't it seem reasonable that some attention be paid to how we maintain and store glucose for the brain? Furthermore, wouldn't it make sense if we had some kind of indicator to let us know when our brains are running low on fuel? To answer those questions, let's consider a parallel reservoir management system.[21]

"Blood sugar measurement does not give us a reliable indication of fuel availability for the brain, except in the very short term (a few minutes at best), just as water flowing from the tap is not a measure of water availability, except in the short term."

Whenever we open the faucet on our sink any given morning, we take for granted that sufficient water reserves will be available for drinking, cooking and other essential activities that we have come to expect with civilized living. As long as water flows, we are content, but in reality we have no indication of the reserve remaining in the reservoir or water tower. In times of drought, that reserve may not be optimal. Without someone to monitor those reserves and warn of limited supply, we would be unlikely to reduce consumption when appropriate. We are blind to actual reserve water supplies.

Our body, with regard to glucose availability and reserves, functions like one turning on the faucet expecting water to flow. It assumes that as long as food intake continues, there will be sufficient supply for the brain. Unfortunately, such is not the case. The body is in effect "blind" to the energy needs of the brain.

Our brain, on the other hand, is like the monitor of the reservoir whose job it is to measure and report on actual water availability. It would be quite foolish and shortsighted, in the extreme, if the brain were to base its fuel availability calculations simply on the supply of glucose available in circulating blood. Doing that is not dissimilar to the assumption we make about our domestic supply of water flowing from the tap on any given day. When the water flows, we assume that there is sufficient supply.

However, isn't that just what physicians and other health professionals do when they order a blood sugar test? Blood sugar measurement does not give us a reliable indication of fuel availability for the brain, except in the very short term (a few minutes at best), just as water flowing from the tap is not a measure of water availability, except in the short term. Both say nothing about the actual status of the reservoir. Just as there are consequences from ignoring the warnings of the water reservoir monitor from our public water department, so are there consequences from ignoring the monitor of the fuel reserve for our brain.

Most of us are unaware that we have a built-in monitor of brain fuel availability or how it works. Don't be surprised; most doctors are unaware of it too. Oh they can tell you what happens when the fuel supply for the brain runs low, and they can describe the consequences of ignoring the warning signs, just as you can. But few, if any, pay any attention to the most important fuel reserve for the brain, nor can they tell you how to maintain it.

Measurement of the one best indicator of brain fuel reserve is not done in routine clinical practice. Yet as we shall see, this indicator is the key to understanding and preventing all the conditions and diseases we know to be associated with the metabolic syndrome – obesity, diabetes, cardiovascular disease, osteoporosis, hypothyroidism, degenerative brain conditions including Alzheimer's disease and even some forms of cancer. We'll come back to this indicator later in Chapter 5.

The human brain is an organ with a colossal demand for fuel (glucose) and yet it has no reserve energy supply. The brain therefore depends on its monitoring and regulatory role to allocate and partition its energy supply. It considers its own demands as "priority one" even to the extent of depriving other organs and tissues of their energy supply when it senses that its supply is running low.

The Fuel Reserves for the Brain

So where does the brain get its fuel? The one source that we have already mentioned is glucose in the circulating blood (blood sugar). The average quantity of blood in the adult human system is around five liters, and each liter will contain around one gram of glucose. This gives us a total blood sugar available at any one time of about five grams. That amount could provide fuel for the brain for about one hour assuming no other organs or tissues were consuming glucose – not a good assumption. In actual life, the blood sugar "reserve" will fuel the brain for no more than a few minutes before the blood glucose concentration drops to a dangerously low level (as in hypoglycemia). Shortly thereafter, a coma would be activated as a desperate last-resort strategy to maintain the life of the brain.

The brain must, therefore, have a more substantial fuel reserve that it may use between meals and during overnight fasting and exercise. This reserve is the liver glycogen store, the only reserve store of glucose that may be released for the brain. The average capacity of this storage reserve is about 75 grams (the range may vary from 60 to 110 grams of glycogen depending on body size and other conditions of overall liver health). Given the fact that the liver will release about 10 grams per hour of glucose during rest to provide fuel for the brain, red blood cells and the kidneys, the liver glycogen reserve will provide enough fuel for the brain for six to eight hours.

The Glycemic Index – A Shortsighted Index that Ignores Brain Fuel Supply

There is no direct way to measure the amount of liver glycogen that remains in storage, except for a rather uncomfortable, invasive (not to mention bloody) liver biopsy, something that is never done for this purpose! And as we have pointed out earlier, a simple measurement of blood glucose would be of limited interest to the brain beyond the succeeding few minutes. An index that measures the blood glucose concentration provided by various foods would therefore be deeply flawed in any application relating to brain fuel or energy reserve. Yet this is exactly what some scientists and nutritionists have done by inventing the glycemic index (GI). The GI is a measure based on a transient value of limited significance. So where did this irrelevant measure come from?

We will describe the GI in more detail in Chapter 4 and only note for now that historically, the glycemic index was developed at the University of Toronto by a group led by Dr. David Jenkins.[22] It was devised as a method of controlling blood glucose concentration for diabetics. The assumption was that individuals with glucose intolerance could ingest certain carbohydrate foods (those with a lower GI) so that glucose would be released into the circulation at a slower rate and thus allow the blood glucose concentration to remain more stable. The intent of consuming low GI foods was to prevent blood glucose concentration from rising that in turn might trigger an excessive release of insulin, a key problem in diabetes.

Focusing on the GI overlooks a more serious probability - brain fuel supply is ignored.

However, as we have stated, the blood glucose measurement is a very transient value. It is not only short term, but also one-dimensional. The result of giving credence to the GI is that a much more serious probability is overlooked. The longer-term glucose supply for the brain is not sufficiently considered or is simply ignored. Furthermore, a much more dangerous short-term possibility is introduced, that of a rapid fall in blood glucose concentration from excessive insulin release following carbohydrate ingestion. This kind of one-dimensional thinking is illustrated by the fact that some believe that a high GI food may be suitable for energy recovery after endurance exercise or for persons experiencing hypoglycemia. While it is certain that a high GI food causes a more rapid rise in blood sugar levels, it is highly questionable that these foods are suitable for exercise recovery.

In the case of a person experiencing an episode of hypoglycemia (or low blood sugar), a high GI food may not be the best option. Hypoglycemia is potentially a very dangerous metabolic situation that threatens glucose supply to the brain and may result, if not resolved rapidly, in a coma. When a glucose (high GI) solution or food is ingested in this situation, a predictable metabolic dynamic would ensue. The glucose is rapidly absorbed from the gastrointestinal tract into the blood stream and immediately raises the blood glucose concentration. Energy is provided for the brain from this circulating glucose. So far, so good.

What follows, however, may not be the most beneficial outcome with respect to ongoing cerebral energy supply. The rapid rise in blood glucose concentration provokes an immediate insulin response. The increased insulin release from the pancreas quickly drives the glucose into muscle and other peripheral tissues, an action that effectively lowers the blood glucose level. Potentially this could lead to another episode of hypoglycemia.

If the liver glycogen store is already depleted (an event that may have triggered the hypoglycemia in the first instance), a further hypoglycemic event is quite likely. Indeed the regulatory response to the first episode may have hastened the liver depletion, increasing the risk of a second episode.

In studies of diabetic patients, it is well known that an episode of hypoglycemia predisposes the subject to later episodes.[23] The ingestion of a lower glycemic index food may actually provide a more long term and stable supply of cerebral energy in such a rapidly developing critical situation, especially if that low GI food were to facilitate the uptake of glucose into the liver. In other words, a lower glycemic index food may be advantageous by virtue of the fact that a portion of the carbohydrate is partitioned not to the circulation, but to the liver where it may be stored for later use.

Foods That Partition Glucose into the Liver

Are there foods that have this remarkable ability to partition glucose away from the blood and into the liver? Yes, but you may be surprised as to which foods can do this. Such foods are those that contain fructose, or fruit sugar, another simple sugar, along with equal amounts of glucose. These foods are fruits, some vegetables and *honey*, or in other words, foods that contain a balanced or nearly equal ratio of glucose to fructose without an excessive amount of starch.

But how can foods containing glucose *and* fructose actually work to lower blood sugar? That seems rather counterintuitive. We have already noted that when starchy foods, which are nothing more than glucose, are ingested, glucose rapidly reaches the circulation prompting a rise in blood glucose along with a release of insulin. But when glucose and fructose are ingested together in nearly equal proportions, something dramatically different happens.

The secret is fructose. Here is how it works. The liver is the primary organ in the body that contains the fructose enzyme, fructokinase. Fructokinase in the liver starts the process whereby fructose is converted to and stored as liver glycogen. Furthermore, fructose, when ingested in the correct ratio with glucose, improves glucose uptake into the liver by acting to liberate the glucose enzyme (glucokinase) from the liver cell nucleus. Glucokinase is necessary for glucose to be converted to and stored as glycogen. Thus fructose is responsible for the creation and storage of glycogen in the liver that serves as the primary energy reserve for the brain.

The Facts about Fructose

There is much conflicting talk about fructose today. Let's sort out what is true from what is exaggeration or myth. As we have indicated, fructose in the diet is essential for glucose to be taken into the liver where it is converted to glycogen and stored. Without fructose, glucose essentially bypasses the liver and raises the blood sugar level causing an insulin spike that drives the glucose into the cells where it is used for energy or stored as muscle glycogen or fat. In other words, fructose is essential in its role as facilitating brain fuel reserve storage.

As a fuel for energy in the rest of the body, fructose is relatively worthless. The muscle cells can't take it in. It cannot be stored in fat cells. Except for the liver, the only other cells in the body that can take in fructose and convert it to glycogen or utilize it for energy are sperm cells, which is a benefit for about half of the population.

In spite of its insignificance in providing fuel for nearly every cell in the body, it is necessary to emphasize the importance of fructose in the diet, especially as it relates to the provision of energy for the brain. Without it, liver glycogen is not rapidly formed, and the brain's energy reserve is not replenished.

"A little fructose is essential. Too much fructose is potentially extremely harmful to your health."

There is, however, a big caution about fructose that must be underscored. There is a limit as to the amount of fructose that can be used by the liver at any one time. As the liver is the only organ in the body that can metabolize small quantities of fructose, excessive amounts of fructose can quickly overwhelm the liver. Once the liver glycogen store is full, no more fructose can be converted and stored as glycogen. And in an attempt to get rid of excessive fructose, the liver simply breaks it down into three-carbon molecules that enter the fatty acid cycle to form triglycerides which combine to form very low density lipoproteins (VLDL) which enter the blood stream and are carried to fat cells for storage.

The amount of fructose consumed by the average American today is in excess of 150 grams (or about one-third of a pound) per day. Multiple research studies over the past 15 years have associated this level of fructose consumption with obesity, elevated triglycerides, cardiovascular disease and diabetes. A recent study has shown that even 74 grams of fructose a day from HFCS (the equivalent to the amount in two and one-half cans of soft drinks or 30 ounces) is associated with high blood pressure.[24]

A little fructose is essential. Too much fructose is potentially extremely harmful to your health. As the liver can only store 75 grams of glycogen at once, a good estimate of the maximum amount of fructose that should be consumed at any one time along with glucose is significantly less than half that amount or about 30 grams (the amount contained in 16 ounces of a soft drink).

As an illustration, a tablespoon of honey (21 grams) contains an average of 7.5 grams of glucose and 8.6 grams of fructose, equivalent to the amounts found in one medium sized apple. This amount of fructose and glucose would result in the formation of about 15 grams of liver glycogen. Two tablespoons of honey would result in the formation of between 25 to 30 grams of liver glycogen, just the right amount to "top-off" the liver glycogen reserve at bedtime or between meals.

This modest amount presents a stark contrast to what happens when one consumes a "Big Gulp®"[25] from your local convenience store. A thirty-two ounce soft drink contains over 75 grams of fructose alone. Along with nearly an equal amount of glucose, this sugar blast forces the liver to metabolize the excess fructose into fatty acids and initiates a massive insulin spike which stores the excess glucose as fat in the muscle and fat cells.

The 13 (Often Ignored) Principles of Fueling the Brain

The preceding information underscores for us a few key principles of brain fueling that merit restating. They have more to do with causality than treating symptoms, and therefore they lead to preventive strategies rather than therapeutics. For some, they may seem counterintuitive. Nevertheless, they are true.

We present them here in summary. Throughout the rest of the book we will describe in detail how these principles can be applied to improving your health. Understanding these principles will help you get beyond the glycemic index in your diet and focus on the more important issue of liver glycogen formation which is "monitored" by the brain fuel indicator or BFI.

They are listed in numerical order, but such listing implies no particular priority. Here they are:

1. Brain (or cerebral) hunger is the driving force behind obesity, diabetes, and all of the conditions and diseases associated with the metabolic syndrome.

2. The brain has no primary fuel reserve of its own and without fuel delivered from the circulating blood brain cells would survive barely 30 seconds.

3. Circulating blood sugar is limited (five to five and one-half grams at any given time) and can only provide enough fuel for the brain for 30 minutes or less.

4. The brain uses glucose as its primary source of energy. The brain will burn amino acids from proteins and some lactic acid but both of these fuels are in short or transient supply in the circulation. Only under limited circumstances does the brain burn fats for energy, such as in the latter stages of starvation and only after blood glucose and liver glycogen stores are exhausted.

5. Though the brain uses glucose as its primary source of energy, excessive glucose consumption (or consumption of foods that are immediately converted to glucose in the digestive process) will not result in adequate brain fueling.

6. The liver is the primary fuel source and active fuel reserve for the brain.

7. The liver forms glycogen from fructose and glucose when these two sugars are ingested together. (The liver also forms glycogen from left over lactic acid or lactate from muscles but this supply is limited. Some glycogen is also produced from amino acids.)

8. When the liver glycogen supply is running low, the liver signals the brain of an impending fuel crisis.

9. The brain responds to this signal by initiating a form of metabolic stress, releasing adrenalin and cortisol from the adrenal glands. Cortisol

is responsible for the breakdown of protein into amino acids that are then carried back to the liver where new glucose is formed (gluco-neogenesis). Adrenalin triggers the release of glycogen from the liver, increases the heart rate and raises blood pressure, insuring that circulation to the liver and brain is maintained.

10. *Metabolic stress* is part of the brain's normal strategy to ensure its own fuel supply first.
11. The brain is a greedy taskmaster, competing for fuel resources with the rest of the body.
12. Factors such as obesity (increased body mass), high levels of lipids in the blood, chronically elevated blood sugar levels, glucose intolerance, and insulin resistance increase the metabolic demand on the body and further deplete the fuel resources needed by the brain for survival.
13. Fueling your liver by consuming fructose / glucose balanced foods (fruits, some vegetables and honey) fuels your brain by allowing for the direct formation of liver glycogen.

Understanding and applying these principles is critical not only for improved health and the reversal of disease progression but also for prevention of disease. It's not too late to get started. Your health depends on it.

Jeanne's Story

Jeanne weighed a scant 100 pounds when she graduated from college at age 21. At age 50 she tipped the scale at more than 150 pounds, a 50% increase in body mass. Throughout the years she complained of episodes of "low blood sugar" (reactive hypoglycemia her doctor called it). Her solution was to carry small containers of peanut butter or bags of nuts or portions of cheese that she consumed whenever she felt lightheaded or shaky. These did little for her early morning symptoms but did temporarily resolve her low blood sugar episodes during the day. As she got older, however she awakened most mornings with waves of nausea and headaches. Her practice was not to eat before bedtime, believing what her mother had told her that eating before bed would only turn to fat. Her morning wake-ups were increasingly distressful.

What may have been a mild annoyance at age 30 now became a major challenge of midlife. It seemed that Jeanne was tired all the time. Her sleep patterns were irregular and punctuated by periods of wakefulness and restlessness. She complained of excessive daytime sleepiness, and weekends were mostly wasted just trying to catch up on rest.

She found it increasingly difficult to concentrate at times and even worried about becoming increasingly forgetful. Her doctor told her she was "pre-diabetic," meaning that her blood sugar was higher than normal. Her lab tests also showed that her thyroid function was low, and her doctor wanted to put her on thyroid supplements, which, he said, would help with her chronic fatigue. Her serum calcium also was low and she was worried about osteoporosis.

Menopausal symptoms were also becoming a major challenge. Her "private summers" were distracting, unsettling, and unpredictable. It was all part of growing old she reasoned, but she was not growing old gracefully.

Attempts to lose weight were cyclical and increasingly futile, typically resulting in short-term loss of a few pounds followed by gaining a few more. She bounced from one diet to another and even tried fasting for 12 hours a day for a time in hopes that the pounds would magically disappear. Instead, everything seemed to get worse. Her weight increased, her sleep patterns became even more irregular. Her chronic tiredness increased. Her menopausal symptoms intensified.

Sound familiar? Jeanne's story is common. She was heading for a metabolic meltdown. She faced a difficult choice - follow her doctor's advice and start taking multiple medicines designated to control her symptoms and modulate her "numbers" or find another way of reversing 30 years of dietary indiscretions and poor lifestyle choices.

Size really matters if you are reaching middle age weighing 50% more than you did at age 21. The reason is quite obvious. Though one's size and weight may have increased significantly with age, the liver's ability to capture and store glycogen has not. If anything, the glycogen storage capacity may decrease with age due to fatty accumulations (excess triglycerides and fatty acids) within the liver cells or liver cell destruction secondary to alcohol consumption or disease.

One's need for glycogen from the liver to fuel the brain, red blood cells and kidneys, as well as a significantly increased body mass, may increase rather dramatically with age. That means that the brain is in competition with the rest of the body for the same energy store. The excess demand for glucose by a now much larger body mass may not be met by readily available glucose. This presents a problem for the brain that depends on a stable and constant energy supply from the liver glycogen reserve.

Jeanne's "meltdown" came in the way of a hypertensive crisis. The emergency physician thought initially that she was having a heart attack because of her presenting chest pain. After testing and observation, it was determined that Jeanne was experiencing the results of chronic metabolic stress. Medication and rest seemed to control the symptoms for a time and Jeanne was given a reprieve.

Chapter 4

Fast Track

- The popular glycemic index (GI) is short sighted and blind to the physiologic complexities of the human system.
- Foods containing fructose will have a lower GI than one with the same amount of other carbohydrates simply because fructose does not contribute to an elevation of blood glucose.
- The limitations of the GI severely compromise its usefulness as a tool in doing anything that is clinically relevant or even practically helpful in any nutritional or dietary sense.
- The limitations of the GI extend to the glycemic load (GL) and the estimated glycemic load (eGL™).
- The logic of using high GI foods after exercise is questionable.

The Glycemic Index

*D*r. David Jenkins and his colleagues at the University of Toronto developed the glycemic index, or GI, in 1981.[26] Their idea was simply to develop a scale for rating foods that were best for individuals with glucose intolerance or diabetes. The GI was created in theory as a way of making sound recommendations for the dietary management of diabetes.

There is "insufficient evidence to support the applicability of the GI or its theory in providing dietary guidelines for glucose intolerance . . ."

Twenty years after Jenkins introduced the GI, attempts to legitimize its use in dietary management, diabetes control, weight loss and general health guidelines continued, specifically from the University of Sydney, Australia, and the work of JC Brand-Miller and her associates. "Despite controversial beginnings, the GI is now widely recognized as a reliable, physiologically based classification of foods according to their postprandial glycemic effect."[27]

Such statements lack credibility, however when viewed from the contemporary understanding of human physiology with regard to brain fueling and the brain energy reserve. More than one hundred scientific studies have been completed in the past 30 years in attempts to define, "calibrate," redefine, or in some way prove the relevance of the GI in dietary guidelines and in the management of blood sugar. A search for "glycemic index" on any internet search engine will result in hundreds of thousands of hits and direct one to dozens of diet plans based on the theory of the GI. In fact, several very popular and successful diet plans

have based their recommendations on the "scientifically proven" GI.[28] Yet, today there remains insufficient
evidence to support the applicability of the GI or its
theory in providing dietary guidelines for glucose
intolerance[29] or weight management for that matter.

It would not be necessary to waste any more ink
on the subject if it were not for the fact that the GI
represents how side-tracked some in the medical and
scientific community have become when it comes to
recommendations for controlling blood sugar and
"treating" glucose intolerance. The GI also illustrates
how a concept that appears to be based on common
sense is in reality very shortsighted or blind to the
physiologic complexities of the human system.

The GI can be defined quite simply as a way to
"measure" the effect of carbohydrates on blood glucose compared to some "standard." Stated that way,
the GI seems reasonable enough. The fact is that the
actual definition of the GI is based on a specific calculation that is too complex for it to be understood by
the average person.[30] Compounding that is the fact
that the standard itself has changed in the years since
the GI was first introduced. For now, we will assume
that the GI of glucose is 100. All other carbohydrate
containing foods will have a GI of some number in
relation to 100, such as those listed in the following
table. (For a more complete listing of the Glycemic
Index (GI) and Glycemic Load (GL) for selected foods,
see Appendix C.)

Glycemic Index and Glycemic Load for Common Foods[31]

Food	GI	Serving Size	Net Carbs	GL
Glucose	100	50 gm	50	50
Peanuts	14	4 oz (113g)	15	2
Grapefruit	25	1/2 large (166g)	11	3
Pizza	30	2 slices (260g)	42	13
Low fat Yogurt	33	1cup (245g)	47	16
Apple	38	1 medium (138g)	16	6
Spaghetti	42	1 cup (140g)	38	16
Carrots	47	1/2 large (72g)	5	2
Orange	48	1 medium (131g)	12	6
Banana	52	1 large (136g)	27	14
Brown Rice	55	1 cup (195g)	42	23
Honey	55	1 Tbsp (21g)	17	9
Oatmeal	58	1 cup (234g)	21	12
Ice cream	61	1 cup (72g)	16	10
Mac & Cheese	64	1 serving (166g)	47	30
Raisins	64	1 small box (43g)	32	20
White Rice	64	1 cup (186g)	52	33
Sugar (sucrose)	68	1 Tbsp (12g)	12	8

Food	GI	Serving Size	Net Carbs	GL
White Bread	70	1 slice (30g)	14	10
Watermelon	72	1 cup (154g)	11	8
Popcorn	72	2 cups (16g)	10	7

There is a bit of truth hidden in the GI value of foods as listed in the above table, but nothing stated in the definition of the GI or in the way in which the GI is applied to nutritional recommendations would reveal that truth. Note the foods listed in the first half of the list following glucose. You can't see it, but all of those contain a higher level of either fructose or protein than those on the last half. The protein content of foods would obviously not contribute directly to an immediate elevation of blood sugar so this is not surprising.

Fructose, even though it is a six-carbon sugar similar to glucose, also does not contribute to an immediate elevation in the blood sugar. Fructose can only be metabolized in the liver where it is either converted to glycogen or broken down into three-carbon chain trioses (a simple three-carbon sugar) that enter into the fatty acid cycle and form triglycerides. Foods that are high in fructose (fruits, some vegetables and honey) would also be expected to have a lower GI than carbohydrates that contain mainly starch or glucose even though their total sugar content might be the same.

So far, so good. Let's summarize:

1. Almost all carbohydrates are metabolized into glucose by the body.
2. Some carbohydrates take longer to be broken down into glucose, thus they take longer to enter the circulation as blood sugar (or blood glucose).
3. The rate at which carbohydrates cause an elevation in blood sugar depends on how quickly they are metabolized (digested).
4. The GI is in theory a methodology for determining the rate at which certain carbohydrates enter the blood and produce a rise in blood sugar.
5. Carbohydrates that have a high GI are broken down into glucose more rapidly, enter the blood quickly and produce a more rapid insulin response.
6. Carbohydrates with a lower GI are broken down more slowly, thereby producing a delayed or more gradual release of glucose into the blood.
7. Fructose containing foods will have a lower GI than one with the same amount of other carbohydrate simply because fructose does not contribute to an elevation of blood glucose.
8. Fructose containing foods will also lower blood glucose by allowing more glucose to be brought into the liver and stored as glycogen.
9. Fructose that is directly converted to and stored as glycogen in the liver will contribute to blood glucose as the liver releases its glycogen supply during times when blood sugar is low.

Now it starts to get a bit more complicated.

The Glycemic Index, Insulin Response and Demand

When glucose reaches the blood, the pancreas responds almost immediately by releasing insulin. The amount of insulin released is usually proportional to the amount of glucose entering the blood (glycemic load). The role of insulin is to drive circulating blood sugar into the cells of the body where it may be used for energy to power the cells in their specific functions.

A food with a lower GI should in theory suggest a lower insulin response or demand, but such is not always the case. In other words, foods that are digested and released into the blood more slowly as glucose should not trigger as high of insulin response as foods that reach the blood more rapidly. If that were always true, a lower GI rated carbohydrate (such as brown rice with a GI of 55) might be recommended as providing better blood sugar control and stability than a high GI rated food (such as white bread with a GI of 70). This assumption also does not take into consideration the total carbohydrate or calorie amount that may vary significantly from food to food. (Note the difference in total carbs between an orange and a banana that have similar GI values, yet a banana has more than twice as many carbs.)

This leads us to several limitations of the GI that severely compromise its usefulness as a tool in doing anything that is clinically relevant or even practically helpful in any nutritional or dietary sense.

Limitations of the Glycemic Index

The limitations of the GI are many. The first is illustrated by the following table that groups foods together in categories depending on their classification as "Low," "Medium" or "High GI."[32]

Classification	GI Range	Examples
Low GI	55 or less	Most fruits and vegetables, legumes, whole grains, meat, eggs, milk, nuts, fructose and other foods low in carbohydrates
Moderate GI	56-69	Whole wheat products, basmati rice, sweet potato, sucrose (table sugar)
High GI	70 and above	Baked potato, watermelon, white bread, most white rice, corn flakes and other breakfast cereals, glucose

As K. Beals points out in her excellent review article on the GI, the "values representing low, moderate, and high GI" foods are "not based on physiological, metabolic, or even statistical rationale."[33] In fact, the cut-off values for certain foods seem to have been arbitrarily determined to insure a variety of foods were included in the "low GI" category.

"These factors all point to a certain unreliability of the GI as a reproducible scientific tool, especially given the fact that measurements of the GI for the

same foods among several laboratories have shown wide variability."

The amount of carbohydrate consumed at any one time has significant effects on the "glycemic response" of the body. For this reason, an arbitrary value of 50 grams of carbohydrate (a little more than two slices of bread) was chosen for the calculation of the GI. Though this amount was convenient and somewhat logical from a statistical perspective, it hardly relates to "real life" eating situations where amounts of carbohydrates consumed at any one time vary widely. Furthermore the bioavailability of carbohydrates, such as in carbs that contain much fiber, or carbs that contain "resistant starch" limits the application of the GI.[34]

The GI of carbohydrate-rich foods can vary greatly depending on a number of other factors including the variety, origin, processing, and preparation of the food, as well as other nutrients that are consumed with the food. Even the time of day that the foods are consumed and the time when the GI is measured will cause variations.[35] For example, mashing potatoes or decreasing the pH of the starch by adding vinegar, as in potato salad, will raise or lower the GI respectively.[36] The GI of potatoes will also be affected significantly by heating (increases GI[37]) or cooling (lowers the GI[38]). Even the type of cooking method (e.g., baking, boiling or microwaving) seems to have an effect on the GI.[39]

These factors all point to a certain unreliability of the GI as a reproducible scientific tool, especially given the fact that measurements of the GI for the same foods among several laboratories have shown wide variability.[40] There is also significant variability of GI between test subjects[41] as well as variability within individuals on different occasions or at different times of day.[42] These all represent confounding factors that render the GI less than "scientific." In fact, given the information presented above, it is a mystery that the GI has any credible following at all in the dietary world.

Additionally, there are other issues that lead one to conclude that the use of the GI in any serious metabolic consideration is extremely limiting and shortsighted. For example, a lower GI value for any given food suggests a slower rate of digestion and absorption of that particular food's carbohydrates, but it says nothing about the mechanism responsible for that lower value. It may be, as we shall discuss later, that the lower GI value is simply due to a partitioning of that carbohydrate into the liver rather than into the blood.

The GI of fructose is quite low for a simple sugar (19 as compared to 100 for glucose) but this has little or nothing to do with its effect on blood sugar but rather on the fact that the liver is the only organ in the body where fructose can be metabolized and converted into glycogen. Furthermore, foods that contain a balanced ratio of fructose to glucose facilitate the storage of liver glycogen by the formation of liver glycogen directly, a fact that actually contributes to the lowering of blood sugar levels.

While a lower GI value for a food usually equates to an improvement in long-term blood glucose control and a reduction in blood lipid formation, such is not always the case. Again, fructose is a prime example. Excessive consumption of fructose (a low GI carbohydrate), as in foods containing high fructose corn syrup (HFCS), always results in an elevation of triglycerides. Again, as the liver is the only organ that can metabolize large amounts of dietary fructose, it breaks down the six-carbon fructose molecule into three-carbon trioses that immediately enter the fatty acid cycle producing an elevation in triglycerides.

Finally, the GI value for a food might be helpful if it showed correlation with the insulin response caused by the ingestion of that food. Again logic and reality do not support one another as certain foods (e.g., lean meats and proteins) cause an insulin response despite there being no carbohydrates present. Other foods cause a disproportionate insulin response relative to their carbohydrate load.

These glaring and significant limitations of the GI can be summarized as follows: [43]

1. *Lack of consistent data.* Determination of the GI requires actual testing with human subjects, which tends to be expensive. It is estimated that only 5% of all foods have actually been tested and thousands of new foods and food products are released each year. Furthermore, similar foods can have widely varying GI values so it is not always possible to estimate the GI of a food within a specific group.

2. *Wide variations in testing results.* The results of measurements of the GI are not precise. Values of the GI vary among foods, among testing labs, and among individuals being tested. Results may even vary depending on the maturity or ripeness of a food or on the method of processing or preparing the food.

3. *Changes in GI when foods are combined.* Foods that contain fiber, protein, or fat will generally reduce the GI value. The GI of a "mixed meal" can be estimated, but this average becomes less accurate as the carbohydrate content decreases.

4. *Differing rates of digestion.* The GI of the same food will vary from person to person and even with the time of day that it is consumed. Also,

the insulin response to foods having the same GI will vary among individuals.

5. ***Bad data leads to bad outcomes***. Blind reliance on the GI as a nutritional guideline can lead to unanticipated or poor outcomes such as over-consumption or failure to provide proper fuel for the brain.

Glycemic Load

The limitations of the GI as summarized above have led to the development and inclusion of another measure of a carbohydrate's theoretical effect on blood sugar. It is called the glycemic load or GL. The GL is a "relative indication of the likelihood of a food" to increase your blood sugar levels. How's that for a specific scientific definition? Again, the theory is that if one could keep the total GL for all foods consumed in a day below some magic number (typically given as 100), that would somehow improve blood sugar control, improve diabetes management and enhance weight loss.

The GL is calculated by the following formula: GL = GI/100 x Net Carbs. In other words, the GL is based on a calculation of the GI, which we have already shown to be highly variable, inconsistent and some-times inaccurate. Now we have another indicator that we are expected to believe is better? The facts just don't add up. The same limitations that apply to the GI must be applied to the GL, as the calculation of the GL first requires determination of the GI.

In order to overcome the inconsistencies and errors built into the GL by virtue of its dependence on the GI, some have gone a step farther with this questionable logic. They have created (and even trademarked) what is called the "Estimated Glycemic Load" or eGL™.[44] The eGL™ is explained by the Nutrition Data folks as follows:

> "By doing a multivariate analysis on the existing glycemic data, Nutrition Data was able to create a mathematical formula that estimates Glycemic Load by comparing the food's levels of commonly known nutrients. This formula was not intended to completely replace traditional Glycemic Load calculations, but it does produce a reasonable estimation when a food's Glycemic Index is unknown."[45]

When we were in school, which was some time ago, formulas that contained spurious data or data that was inconsistent, unreliable or just plain wrong were themselves no less inconsistent, unreliable or just plain wrong. Have things changed that much today? Even the so-called "benefits" of the eGL™ as stated on NutritionData.com make little sense: "The average diet contains many foods for which Glycemic Index values have not yet been determined. By using eGL to estimate Glycemic Loads for these foods, you receive more complete dietary feedback than if the effects of such foods were simply ignored."[46]

Even if that last statement could be understood (which remains in question), it seems to be saying that knowing *something* is better than knowing *nothing*. But for what purpose and to what result, except that one receives "more complete dietary feedback," whatever that is.

The GI and Recovery after Exercise

Earlier, it was mentioned that a food with a high GI would be highly questionable as a suitable food for recovery following exercise. A qualification is in order. There is actually nothing harmful with using foods with a high GI value following exercise as they certainly do contribute to replenishing muscle glycogen, an important aspect of muscle recovery. This approach, however, ignores the more critical aspect of liver uptake, liver glycogen storage and the provision and maintenance of an ongoing energy supply for the brain.

The availability of a reserve energy supply for the brain is of utmost significance with respect to total body recovery in the post-exercise period. Without sufficient cerebral energy reserve, the brain will initiate a form of metabolic stress to ensure an ongoing fuel supply for itself. Thus, the metabolic stress produced by exercise itself will be compounded, and recovery throughout the body will be delayed pending restored fuel resources for the brain.

During exercise, contracting muscles extract glucose from the circulation. When exercise is prolonged, liver glycogen stores are depleted as more glucose is released into the blood for extraction by the muscles. Thus the contribution of liver glycogen as a fuel for exercise is greater relative to the amount of muscle glycogen derived from within the muscle itself.

This observation is in itself somewhat contradictory, and a brief explanation is needed. Usually insulin is required to transport glucose into muscle cells, as is the case after a meal. However, exercise suppresses insulin release. Therefore, insulin has little active part in the muscle uptake of glucose during exercise.

Muscles overcome this challenge by using a very sophisticated system of transporting glucose across the cell walls. As the muscle cells contract, the glucose transport proteins are driven to the cell wall where they activate the transport of glucose across the cell membrane into the cell itself. Glucose is now available for energy for ongoing muscle cell contractions.

This exercise-induced strategy for powering contracting muscles continues well into the post-exercise period and remains active for several hours after the exercise is finished. Athletes are frequently advised to consume high GI foods during this period in order to maximize muscle uptake of glucose and therefore optimize replenishment of muscle glycogen. As in the case of hypoglycemia, however, described earlier in Chapter 3, this recommendation ignores the issue of provision of energy for the brain.

Given the fact that the provision of energy for the brain is the first priority of metabolism, especially during the recovery phase after exercise, the brain will act in its own interests to ensure its own fuel supply during this time. The mechanism the brain uses to insure fuel for itself is mediated by the hypothalamus-pituitary-adrenal (HPA) axis.[47]

Normally, in the post-exercise period, the HPA axis is calmed or in a state of relative rest. Ingestion of a high GI carbohydrate food or beverage following exercise will induce a potent insulin response which begins partitioning glucose into muscle cells as opposed to leaving it in the circulation for uptake by the brain. In addition, the exercise-induced transport of glucose into the muscle cells remains active, thus providing muscles with two separate systems to maximize the partitioning of glucose into muscle tissue. Thus in the post-exercise period, the muscle cells are rapidly absorbing glucose from the blood stream using two separate methods to do so.

The rapid depletion of liver glycogen during exercise would have resulted in a reduced reserve energy supply available to provide for ongoing energy requirements of the brain. This would have resulted in a signal from the liver to the brain alerting it to the impending fuel shortage. That signal (IGFBP-1) inhibits the actions of another hormone (IGF-1) most responsible for recovery and rebuilding of tissues worn down or damaged by exercise.

The result is not difficult to predict. The HPA axis is reactivated at a time when it should remain in a state of rest. This untimely reactivation of metabolic stress results in the inhibition of recovery physiology. Recovery is compromised and will remain so until the liver glycogen stores are replenished and the brain is satisfied that its fuel supply is sufficient and stable.

Recovery is mediated by the brain and is accompanied by a hormonal cascade (including IGF-1 and growth hormone) affecting all parts of the body. The release of these recovery hormones is absolutely dependent on the ongoing provision of cerebral energy. The overriding metabolic consideration from the perspective of the brain is that of having sufficient energy provision specifically from the liver glycogen reserve.

The most appropriate food to be consumed in the immediate post-exercise period would be a carbohydrate containing a balance of fructose and glucose. Foods such as fruits or fruit juices or honey would be the ideal choices. The GI value for these is actually quite irrelevant. The GI will vary widely depending on the fructose/glucose ratio. The important factor is the ability of these foods to form liver glycogen rapidly and keep the production and release of IGFBP-1 low, thus eliminating or reducing the trigger for metabolic stress.

Perhaps a more relevant indicator of metabolic health would be one that ranks the ability of a food to form liver glycogen based on its relative fructose content. In other words, the liver glycogen "yield" from the ingestion of certain foods would be a better indicator of metabolic health.

In the recipes and menus at the end of this book, we have provided just such a calculation. The amount of liver glycogen expected to be produced from the consumption of particular foods is calculated in **Appendix A**.

Chapter 5

Fast Track

- The brain fuel indicator (BFI) is a protein produced by the liver that warns the brain of an impending low fuel status.
- The BFI is the metabolic equivalent of the low fuel light on your car's instrument panel.
- The BFI is inversely related to liver glycogen levels and rises in proportion to cortisol levels.
- Ignoring liver glycogen and failing to stock the primary brain fuel reserve is called "liver blindness."
- Liver glycogen depletes at the rate of 10 grams per hour at rest which means that the brain's fuel tank only contains enough fuel for about 8 hours, not enough to get through the night if one's last meal was at 6:00 PM.

The Brain Fuel Indicator (BFI) and Its Potential

*J*ust what is the *brain fuel indicator*? For starters, you would not find it by that name in any physiology textbooks. It is not a diagnostic test that your doctor would routinely order. However elusive or unknown this BFI may be, it is nevertheless real.

The BFI is the first and perhaps the most important indicator of metabolic stress in the human body. It is the early warning signal to the brain that its fuel supply is running low.

In biochemical terms, the BFI is a protein produced by the liver known as insulin-like growth factor binding protein-1 or IGFBP-1 for short.[48] It is a protein that works as an endocrine hormone to either inhibit the action of or prolong the half-life of insulin-like growth factor or IGF-1.[49]

"The BFI is actually the earliest stress indicator . . . the metabolic equivalent of the low fuel light on your car's instrument panel."

In the late 1990s, there was a debate in the scientific community over what influenced the release of IGFBP-1. Some believed that an increase in blood plasma cortisol level was the key factor accounting for an increase of IGFBP-1. Others held that a fall in insulin was the major factor prompting the release of this hormone.

It was a study by Jean Marc Lavoie and his team at the University of Montreal in 2002 that settled the debate. Their research showed that IGFBP-1 release was directly related to falling liver glycogen levels. Lavoie's research confirmed that IGFBP-1 is the index of liver glycogen plenitude or status and therefore is the measure of cerebral energy reserve. From the perspective of the "selfish brain," IGFBP-1 is the most critical energy index in metabolism. This is the energy index we refer to as the BFI. We have named it that because of its role in indicating the relative amount of liver glycogen stored in the liver cells as reserve fuel for the brain. When liver glycogen levels are high, the amount of IGFBP-1 produced and released from the liver is low. When liver glycogen is low, IGFBP-1 is high.

The BFI is actually the earliest stress indicator. It alerts the brain when the liver glycogen reserve reaches low levels. It is the metabolic equivalent of the "low fuel" light on your car's instrument panel. The brain responds by triggering the release of stress hormones, cortisol and adrenalin, from the adrenal glands. These stress hormones facilitate the production of new glucose from muscle protein and thus insure an adequate brain fuel supply.

The Key to Understanding Glucose Regulation

It was during the mid 1990s that the importance of a variable metabolic strategy of controlling blood sugar and regulating insulin resistance began to be understood. The key that opened this understanding was the discovery of the relationship between IGFBP-1 (the **BFI**) and liver glycogen levels, blood glucose levels, insulin and cortisol levels and the time of day.[50, 51]

As liver glycogen levels decrease, either in response to the nighttime fast or to prolonged exercise, IGFBP-1 levels in the circulation were increase (See **Approximate Levels of Liver Glycogen / IGFBP-1 / Cortisol** graph below). This triggers the brain to activate the HPA axis to initiate the production of new glucose. IGFBP-1 levels rise, parallel with levels of cortisol, and are inversely related to levels of blood glucose and insulin. As blood glucose and insulin levels increase, the BFI decreases.

[**NOTE**: Unit levels of glycogen, IGFBP-1 and cortisol are relative to each other as shown on the graph. Values given are representative.]

Approximate Levels of Liver Glycogen/IGFBP-1/Cortisol

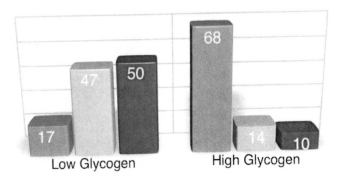

The simplicity of this is really quite astounding. When liver glycogen levels are high (as when the liver glycogen store is full), the BFI and cortisol levels are low. Blood sugar and insulin levels are stable. When liver glycogen levels are low, such as during exercise or during sleep when liver glycogen has not been stored in reserve, the BFI and cortisol levels are increased. The net effect is a form of insulin resistance that blocks glucose from getting into the cells allowing the blood sugar to remain elevated.

This information allows us to understand the mechanism by which the brain is able to regulate the partitioning and provision of fuel for its own needs. The brain depends on input from the liver (the BFI) to know just when to begin allocating fuel for itself. From the perspective of the brain and its energy supply, these are perfectly consistent metabolic events.

The brain works to protect and preserve its own fuel supply above all else. As blood glucose levels decrease, either because of the passage of time since last food intake or by exercise, which accelerates glucose utilization, liver glycogen levels are expected to decrease in an attempt to keep blood glucose stable. The brain is warned of this impending fuel shortage by the BFI and takes immediate action to preserve and increase the amount of circulating glucose.

The fact that the BFI is not yet a standard lab test used in medical practice today may lead one to conclude that it is theoretical or less than important. After all, don't physicians test for about everything that can be measured in attempts to diagnose every other ailment that plagues us?

Liver Blindness

There are, perhaps, reasons why the medical profession, including nutrition experts, dietary gurus and just about everyone else do not know of the BFI. It is not the case that information is lacking about the liver and its critical role in fueling the brain and initiating metabolic stress. Rather it appears that this information has been overlooked or ignored for decades. This *liver blindness*[52] is not a disease as such, but it may be termed a social or cultural disorder, which begins in the medical faculties of our universities, infects other health, nutrition and dietetics institutions, and ultimately impacts the health of generations.

"You may think that you are consuming an appropriate amount of calories. In reality you may not be providing adequate liver glycogen to fuel the brain . . ."

The focus on counting calories or carbohydrate consumption (a "symptom" co-equal with liver blindness with regard to its effects) without regard to the partitioning and the provisioning of those calories as orchestrated by the brain for its own needs, ignores a basic tenant of healthy metabolism. For example, you may think that you are consuming an appropriate amount of calories for your metabolic needs. In reality, you may not be providing timely or appropriate food intake necessary to store adequate liver glycogen to fuel the brain during exercise or during rest. Metabolic stress or activation of the HPA axis as a protective regulatory strategy is the inevitable outcome.

The unfortunate result of activating metabolic stress night after night is an increased risk for all the conditions and diseases associated with the metabolic syndrome. The critical fuel supply depot for the brain has been ignored! Failure to consider the liver and its role in glycogen storage and provisioning is a monumental oversight in contemporary medicine.

The Key to Understanding the Brain Fuel Indicator

The best way to become aware of your own BFI is pay attention to your body. What time do you typically go to bed? Are you eating foods with a balance of fructose and glucose in order to form liver glycogen? What time did you eat those foods? How long before bedtime? What time do you first awaken in the morning? Do you wake up in the early morning hours and have a difficult time getting back to sleep? Is your sleep restful or do you awaken feeling like you have been on a treadmill all night? Answering those questions will give you a good start in understanding the fuel status reserve of the brain - the liver glycogen store.

The graph entitled Liver Glycogen in Grams versus Time indicates what is happening to your liver glycogen levels during the night. From this, we can draw conclusions about what you might need to do that will help you sleep better. Keep in mind that liver glycogen levels do not necessarily correspond to blood sugar levels. Though the body's regulatory mechanisms work hard to keep blood sugar within a fairly narrow range (70 to 110 mg%), blood sugar is transient.

If we were to graph the BFI over the hours of the night in a similar manner, the values for the BFI (IGFBP-1) would be opposite to those for liver glycogen. In other words, BFI is inversely proportional to liver glycogen. When liver glycogen is high as in the early hours of the night, BFI is low. When liver glycogen is low as morning approaches, BFI is high.

Liver Glycogen in Grams versus Time

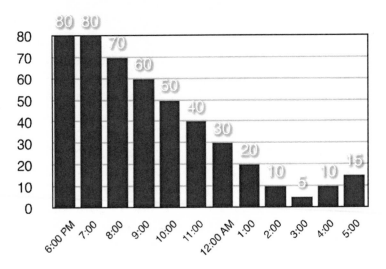

Time - 6:00 PM to 5:00 AM

Note: This graph indicates the approximate levels of liver glycogen following a meal at 6:00 PM. Approximate levels are shown for the next 11 hours assuming no food intake after 6:00 PM and a normal liver glycogen depletion rate. The total amount of glycogen in the liver at any given time is highly variable. Estimates of total glycogen range from 55 to 120 grams depending on body size. Liver glycogen depletion rates also will vary depending on activity and demand. At rest, the liver glycogen store will deplete at a rate of about 10 grams per hour providing 6.5 grams for the brain and 3.5 grams for the kidneys and red blood cells. As liver glycogen levels approach zero, IGFBP-1 is released to signal the brain of an imminent fuel shortage. The brain responds by triggering metabolic stress that promotes formation of new glucose (gluconeogenesis).

Jack's Story

*J*ack was a "jock." From early youth he loved sports, all sports, and he excelled in all of them. He lettered in high school football and baseball. He ran track. He was recruited for college football and eventually became a star running back for his alma mater.

After college, Jack went on to law school, passed the bar exam and entered a law practice. Eventually he became a successful corporate attorney.

Over the years, frequent travel and hours behind the desk cut into his time for athletics and his routine began to include more after-hours socializing than gym time. And though he worked out less and eventually had to curtail his time for exercise entirely, his voracious, high calorie appetite necessary to fuel his exercise regimen of earlier days remained about the same. While he did not gain much weight and continued to look trim and fit, he was shocked to find out during a routine executive physical exam that he was diabetic. He was only 52! How was this possible?

Several factors contributed to his untimely diagnosis. The first had its origins in his teen years. (Metabolic stress and chronic nocturnal cerebral starvation are no respecter of persons or age.) Poor fueling during exhaustive training and athletic performance exacted a toll even though Jack was unaware of it until years later.

Sleep depravation and disrupted sleep patterns compounded his chronic metabolic stress throughout midlife. Poor nutritional habits, which included skipping breakfast and relying on caffeine and donuts, irregular meals, and failure to top off his liver glycogen (brain fuel) reserve before bedtime, kept his adrenalin and cortisol levels unnecessarily high throughout the day and night. As a result, insulin resistance developed and abnormal glucose metabolism ensued.

For years, and perhaps decades, the resiliency of our bodies to internal stress allows us to function without apparent signs or symptoms. Eventually, something gives out. The unfortunate reality is that something is giving out more frequently and much earlier, it seems, than it used to. So it was with Jack. The seeds of metabolic discontent are sown during youth and the fruit matures in midlife.

Chapter 6

Fast Track

- The energy demands of a healthy brain are 20 times greater, gram-for-gram, than the rest of the body.
- The primary fuel reserve for the brain is small (only 75 grams) and must be replenished frequently.
- At rest, the fuel supply for the brain will last seven to eight hours. During intense exercise, the fuel supply will last less than one hour.
- The best strategy for refilling the brain's fuel tank is to consume foods that contain equal amounts of fructose and glucose (honey, fruits and some vegetables) that rapidly restock glycogen in the liver.
- The critical times to fill up the brain's fuel tank are at bedtime, on awakening in the morning, before, during, and after exercise.

The Energy Demands of a Healthy Brain

*T*he brain burns glucose almost exclusively. Compared to other organs or tissues in the body, the brain has a voracious appetite for glucose. In the introduction to the paper "The Selfish Brain, Competition for Energy Resources," Professor Achim Peters of the "Selfish Brain Group" of Germany states:

> ". . . the energy consumption of the brain, related to its small proportion of the entire body mass, is much larger than the energy consumption of all other organs (e.g., muscle). The proportion of energy consumed by the human brain exceeds the proportion found in all other known species . . ."[53]

The colossal energy demand of the brain compared to all other body tissues can be illustrated by the following simple calculations. The human brain uses around 30 Calories (or kilocalories) per hour, or 720 Calories (kilocalories) every 24 hours. An adult weighing 75 Kilograms (165 pounds) would require an average total daily energy expenditure of over 24 hours of about 2500 Calories.

The brain itself weighs about 1500 grams (1.5 Kilogram). Dividing 720 Calories by 1500 grams indicates that the energy expenditure of the brain is 0.48 Calories per gram per 24 hours.

Energy expenditure of the brain per 24 hours:

720 Calories / 1500 grams =
0.48 Calories per gram per day

The remaining 73.5 Kilograms of body mass would consume the remaining 1780 Calories over the 24 hour period. Dividing 1780 Calories by 73500 grams (the weight of the rest of the body not counting the brain) indicates that the energy expenditure for the rest of the body is an average of 0.024 Calories per gram of body tissue over the 24-hour cycle.

Energy expenditure of the rest of the body per 24 hours:

1780 Calories / 73500 grams =
0.024 Calories per gram per day

Each gram of the brain expends 0.48 Calories while each gram of the body expends 0.024 Calories in any 24-hour cycle. That's energy expenditure 20 times greater on a gram-for-gram basis between the brain and the rest of the body!

Yet as has been stated in **Chapter 1**, a diet rich in glucose alone does not and cannot fuel the brain properly even though the brain uses primarily glucose for energy. Though this may seem to be counter-intuitive, it is a metabolic reality. Glucose simply raises blood sugar levels prompting a huge insulin response that drives glucose into the cells and out of reach of the brain.

"It is therefore essential that the major fuel reserve for the brain, the liver glycogen store be replenished frequently."

Since the brain itself does not have a fuel reserve of its own, where does the brain get the amount of fuel required for its energy needs? There are two primary sources for glucose to fuel the brain, the glucose circulating in the blood as blood sugar and the glucose stored in the liver as glycogen. At any given time the amount of glucose in the blood is between five and six grams, enough for about 30 minutes of brain function.

The Brain's Fuel Reserve Needs Frequent Replenishing

The liver glycogen reserve in the average-sized person contains 75 to 80 grams of glucose or enough for about 7 to 8 hours during rest. During intense exercise, this amount of glucose may be enough for only 45 minutes of conscious brain function.

It is therefore essential that the major fuel reserve for the brain, the liver glycogen store, be replenished frequently. This is all the more so when one engages in prolonged exercise and most certainly before sleep, a period when the brain risks being deprived of fuel if the liver glycogen reserve runs low.

How then does one best provide for the energy requirements of the brain? And how often do these requirements need to be met to avoid the initiation of metabolic stress? The answer of course depends on the status of the liver glycogen reserve and on the foods selected throughout the day to restock liver glycogen levels. As indicated previously, the liver will release an average of 10 grams of glycogen each hour during rest to provide energy for the brain, kidneys and red blood cells. During intense exercise, as much as 100 grams per hour may be released from the liver, which means that new glucose would have to be formed during exercise just to keep up with the needs of the brain, kidneys and red blood cells and the exercising muscles.

Dietary Options for Fueling the Brain

The options for fueling the brain are now becoming clearer. One option might be to consume glucose rich carbohydrates continuously (or at least every 30 minutes) throughout the day to keep the blood sugar levels constant as blood glucose is one of the sources for brain fuel.

This, however, would be a treacherous plan of action with disastrous results and severe negative health consequences. The insulin response would continually be challenged to release more and more insulin, which would drive more glucose into the cells, dropping the blood glucose level to dangerously low levels and initiating metabolic stress. Activity levels would typically not be sufficient throughout the day to burn the excessive amounts of glucose being consumed, so most of it would be stored as fat within the muscle and fat cells. Eventually, insulin resistance would develop and some level of glucose intolerance would follow.

You can imagine the outcome of a few weeks or months of following this plan. Yet this is exactly the strategy followed by a large percentage of our population who frequently indulge in carbohydrates from beverages and other sweets during most awake hours of the day. True, there are differences of degree or scale or length of time that this strategy is in play. But the outcome is eventually the same.

A variation of this ill-fated strategy is one suggested by physicians to folks who suffer from reactive hypoglycemia or low blood sugar. These individuals are encouraged to consume some protein snacks such as nuts or peanut butter or cheese, along with carbohydrates to get their blood sugar back to normal. While it is true that proteins will eventually be broken down into amino acids that can be converted to glucose in the liver, this process may take a couple of hours or more under normal conditions. The new glucose formed in the liver will then be released into the blood.

A similar event occurs with low GI foods that take longer to be digested into glucose and absorbed into the blood. Yet, both proteins and low GI foods will do little or nothing to correct the underlying problem, low liver glycogen levels.

"The best strategy for fueling the brain involves consuming foods that rapidly form liver glycogen . . . foods that contain equal or nearly equal portions of glucose and fructose, honey, fruits and most vegetables."

The best strategy for fueling the brain involves consuming foods that rapidly form liver glycogen, the primary fuel reserve for the brain. These are foods that contain equal or nearly equal portions of glucose and fructose - honey, fruits and most vegetables.

Most of us have heard that a healthy diet should consist of five servings of fruits and vegetables a day. The advice sounds good. Yet even the nutritionists and dietitians who make such recommendations would not relate it to the need for producing liver glycogen to fuel the brain.

The Critical Times to Restock Liver Glycogen

As has been said, there are two periods during which the liver glycogen reserve would be expected to be low, early in the morning, or any other time when one has gone without food for several hours, and following prolonged exercise (lasting 45 minutes or more). During sleep, liver glycogen would have been depleted to fuel the brain, kidneys and red blood cells. After exercise, the same would be true.

From this we suggest that the most logical times to replenish liver glycogen are the following:

- Just before bedtime
- On awakening in the morning
- Before and during exercise lasting more than an hour
- After exercise

Before Bedtime

The reason that it is critical to top off the liver glycogen reserve before bedtime is that most of us eat our last meal of the day around 6:00 PM and avoid eating anything before bedtime, believing the myth that food consumed before bed will just turn to fat. Even if our evening meal contained a good fructose-glucose balance, by 10:00 or 11:00 PM our liver glycogen reserve may be half-depleted, leaving only enough glycogen for 3 or 4 hours of uninterrupted sleep.

We have said that the best strategy for ensuring an adequate liver glycogen store overnight is of course to eat foods that contain both fructose and glucose (fruits, some vegetables and honey), but consuming fiber-laden fruits and excessive carbs from vegetables may not be the best strategy, especially during a time when the GI tract is powering down for the night. Honey, on the other hand, is the ideal food to provide energy for the brain during the night's fast. When consumed before bedtime, honey replenishes the liver glycogen store providing enough brain fuel for 7 to 8 hours of restful sleep.[54] Honey contains a nearly equal balance of fructose and glucose. Each tablespoon of honey (21 grams) contains an average of 7.5 grams of glucose and 8.6 grams of fructose plus two or three other complex sugars (polysaccharides) in small amounts. When consumed by itself, a tablespoon of honey would provide 64 Calories and produce about 15 to 17 grams of liver glycogen.[55] Two tablespoons of honey would provide 30 grams of liver glycogen or more than one-third the total capacity of the liver.

"The ingestion of an ounce of honey (about two tablespoons) in the late evening hours before bedtime will ensure that the liver glycogen store will be full so that restful uninterrupted sleep and recovery physiology can occur."

Can one consume too much honey? As the liver is the only organ in the body that can metabolize fructose, six tablespoons of honey, for example, or about one-third of a cup, would present the liver with more fructose (and glucose) at one time than it can possibly take in and store. When confronted with such an excessive amount of fructose, the liver stops everything else that it is doing to digest the fructose. It does this by breaking down the six-carbon chain molecule of fructose into two three-carbon molecules or trioses, which are converted to triglycerides or fats.

The ingestion of an ounce of honey (about two tablespoons) in the late evening hours before bedtime will ensure that the liver glycogen store will be full so that restful uninterrupted sleep and recovery physiology can occur. The primary reasons for this are simple and straightforward:

- Honey packs a dense caloric load, that is, a small amount provides a relatively large amount of energy.
- Honey presents the gut with a low digestive burden as honey contains no fiber to speak of and very little mass for such a high caloric load. Absorption into the blood stream is rapid leaving the GI tract quiet for the night.
- Honey ingestion, with its nearly equal portions of fructose and glucose, results in immediate formation of liver glycogen that fuels the brain during the night fast.
- Honey is a high-octane fuel providing more liver glycogen per gram than any other food.

A well-fueled brain is a contented brain, able to orchestrate the events of recovery and restoration during sleep without interruption and without initiating metabolic stress to secure additional energy supplies for itself.

Fruits and juices would be acceptable foods for consumption just before bedtime except for the water content. The amount of liver glycogen produced by a cup (8 ounces) of juice would be expected to be nearly the same as from a tablespoon of honey, but the disadvantages are more marked when the doses are doubled. To get the same amount of liver glycogen as from two tablespoons of honey, one would have to drink two cups of juice. This probably would be an excessive amount of liquid for most to consume just before bedtime.

The primary goal of this late night refueling is again to produce enough liver glycogen to fuel the brain for 8 hours of sleep. A full liver glycogen reserve will do this for just about everyone. When liver glycogen is adequate, less IGFBP-1 is produced in the liver to warn the brain of impending fuel shortage. When IGFBP-1 is kept low, less cortisol and adrenaline will be released, meaning that more restful sleep is possible.

On Awakening

Unless you make a habit of raiding the refrigerator between 3:00 and 4:00 AM each morning, you will awaken around 7:00 AM with a liver almost totally depleted of glycogen. Some of you may recognize this as hypoglycemia. You may even be nauseated, as in "morning sickness" but you don't have to be pregnant to experience this. It happens to nearly everyone at some time.

Early morning nausea is caused in part by the secretion of glucagon from the pancreas. Glucagon, a hormone that has the opposite effect to insulin, raises blood sugar levels and causes the liver to convert its glycogen into glucose so that it can be released into the blood. Early in the morning, there may not be much liver glycogen left in reserve.

IGFBP-1 levels would be elevated and the brain would have triggered the onset of metabolic stress, releasing more adrenalin and cortisol that result in feelings of shakiness or headache. Because of the nausea, the temptation is to skip breakfast or simply grab a cup of coffee and pastry on the way to work.

"The first meal of the day is not the time to overdo it with carbohydrates that only contain excessive amounts of simple sugars, sucrose or HFCS . . . the goal is to replenish the depleted liver glycogen store, not just raise your blood sugar levels."

A breakfast consisting mainly of carbohydrates, such as cereal, pastries, donuts, or toast and jam is one of the poor dietary habits followed by most of us since our youth. These carbohydrate-rich foods are broken down rapidly into glucose and absorbed into the blood, causing an immediate elevation in blood glucose. High levels of blood glucose trigger the release of excessive amounts of insulin that quickly drives the glucose into the cells and out of the reach of the brain. Little or no new glycogen will have been formed in the liver. In an hour or two, blood glucose levels will have fallen to low levels triggering another round of metabolic stress producing more cortisol and adrenalin release.

The first meal of the day is not the time to overdo it with carbohydrates that only contain excessive amounts of simple sugars, sucrose or HFCS. Cereals (almost all of them), pastries, donuts, toast with jam, and pancakes or waffles laden with corn syrups should be routinely avoided or eliminated altogether. All of these foods contain too much sugar or HFCS or result in excessive glucose loads after digestion, which rapidly raises blood sugar levels, causing a huge spike in insulin, forcing the quick storage of glucose within the muscle or fat cells as opposed to the liver.

A better option would be to recognize that many of the early morning symptoms of nausea, headache, shakiness and fuzzy thinking come from low blood sugar and a depleted liver glycogen reserve. In spite of the nausea and loss of appetite, the best food to ingest at this time is something that will quickly restore the liver glycogen reserve and stabilize blood sugar.[56]

Breakfast, the first fuel stop of the day should focus on one thing - restoring the liver glycogen reserve, which will be nearly depleted in the early morning hours. If you are diabetic and routinely check your blood sugar in the morning on arising, don't let an elevated reading fool you. This is known as the "dawn phenomenon."

Breakfast is a good time to get additional protein. Eggs, cheese, lean meat or even fish may also be eaten at this time. Don't worry about the cholesterol in egg yolks or dairy products. Many studies have debunked the myth that eating eggs will raise your cholesterol. In fact, what really happens when you consume too much dietary cholesterol is that your body just stops making additional cholesterol for a while until the amount from dietary intake is used up.

Milk is fine (unless you are lactose intolerant) as long as it is not skim milk or non-fat milk. The small amount of fat in milk or 2% milk, like the cholesterol in eggs, is not harmful and will not drive up your cholesterol. Milk contains lactose, a sugar that is made up of galactose and glucose. Galactose, like the fructose in fruits or honey, facilitates the formation of glucose in the liver into glycogen by unlocking the enzyme, glucokinase, from the liver cell nucleus.

Pure fruit juices (not the fruit drinks that have added sugar or HFCS) are a good way to ensure immediate liver glycogen formation. A glass of pure fruit juice or a tablespoon of honey will do the trick. Since one is less concerned about an active gastrointestinal tract in the morning hours, consuming whole fruits at this hour is also a good idea. The list of options is nearly endless and as varied as the seasonal availability.

A cup (8 ounces) of pure orange, apple, or cranberry juice or similar juices prepared from concentrate would contain an average of 20 to 25 grams of sugars, nearly equally divided between fructose and glucose. In general, most fruits will have slightly more glucose than fructose, some more than others. A cup of these juices will provide between 110 and 120 calories. Compared to a tablespoon of honey with 21 grams of sugar (and only 64 calories), these juices provide nearly twice the caloric load and significantly more water that may be a concern for some if consumed before bedtime. That's why breakfast may be a better time for fruits and juices that contain 80 to 90% water.

Tomato juice is slightly different. One cup (240 grams) contains about 10.3 grams of carbohydrates of which 3.7 and 3.3 grams are fructose and glucose respectively, plus nearly two-thirds a gram of sucrose. This amount of tomato juice produces about 41 Calories of energy. In other words, tomato juice has about one-half of the carbs and only one-third as many calories as orange juice, which may be a good thing if one wants to limit calorie intake or reduce weight.

What about whole fruits rather than juices? One small apple contains about the same amount of sugars as one tablespoon of honey. One banana (about one cup) would contain 10 and 11 grams of fructose and glucose respectively and another 12 grams of starch (which we have described earlier as multiple glucose molecules that are joined together) for a total caloric load of over 200 calories.

Watermelon, when in season, is another fruit that contains both fructose and glucose but in different ratios than other fruits or honey. One cup of watermelon contains 11.6 grams of carbohydrate, only about one-half as much as a tablespoon of honey. Yet, this amount of watermelon has only a little over 5 grams of fructose and only 2.4 grams of glucose, plus nearly 2 grams of sucrose and other sugars. The calorie load (46 Calories) for this amount of watermelon is similar to honey.

All fruits and fruit juices contain vitamins and other small amounts of minerals as well as some small amounts of protein, but our discussion here is primarily related to the ability of foods to replenish the depleted liver glycogen store, something that occurs when there is a balance of fructose and glucose.

Before and During Exercise

Since exercise will result in up to 100 grams of glycogen being released from the liver each hour, it is critical that the liver glycogen reserve be topped off *before* exercise and replenished to the extent possible *during* exercise. This is especially true for recreational and professional athletes who work out for long periods during the day or for participants in the extreme sports, e.g., marathons, ultra-marathons, and triathlons, etc. Failure to do so risks the initiation of metabolic stress by a fuel-starved brain during the exercise protocol.

"All exercise poses a threat to the brain."

The timing of fueling before exercise is profoundly related to the timing of the previous meal. Optimally, it is best to eat around 3 hours before exercise to allow time for digestion and storage of fuels. A small snack may be eaten around 90 minutes before beginning an exercise protocol, some cereal with fruit or fruit with honey. Then, it is a good idea to top off the liver with fruit juice or honey 15 to 30 minutes before a race or a workout. This last fueling protocol takes into account liver depletion during the last hour or so before the workout.

All exercise poses a threat to the brain. The brain must constantly legislate between fuel supply to contracting muscles and preserving its own metabolic life. This is precisely why there is confusion in the sport's literature about the adrenal hormones. These hormones (adrenalin and cortisol) limit glucose uptake into contracting muscles during such "fight or flight" episodes, and typically this is the only consideration given to them. Adrenal hormones are actually released to protect fuel supply to the brain. They are neuro-protective hormones. Therefore, if your race lasts 10 seconds or over 10 hours, liver glycogen reserve must be factored into your fueling protocols, before, during, and after exercise, as well as during recovery.

Fueling during exercise and/or participation in sports is obviously going to be somewhat dependent on the sport undertaken. Clearly it is possible to fuel during endurance exercise on a bike as you can easily carry fuel with you, but other protocols such as swimming, running, and skiing present the athlete with challenges. Regardless of the sport, the key is to fuel to whatever maximum when possible.

Until recent years most sport energy drinks were based on glucose and/or glucose polymers that are metabolized rapidly into glucose. Fructose was panned in the literature for several reasons. In the concentrations initially used in studies, fructose caused gut distress. These concentrations were actually much higher than what is found in natural foods. The fructose found in foods is most always balanced with glucose. Furthermore, because muscle cells did not take up fructose during exercise, it was not considered as effective for muscle fueling as glucose.

This view was in line with the general perspective of liver blindness, which was and remains prevalent in sports. In recent years, however, there has been an increased interest in fructose as a fuel. Sport or exercise fuels can now be found that contain fructose along with glucose and/or glucose polymers (chains of repeated glucose units).

With any moderate intensity exercise protocol, the optimum strategy is to rehydrate up to 1 liter per hour and to include with this around 60 grams of carbohydrate. This carbohydrate should include a balance of glucose and fructose (up to a total of 40%) and the rest maltodextrins, complex sugars made up of many glucose molecules linked together. In practical terms, this represents about 2 tablespoons of honey every hour. In longer endurance protocols, energy bars and gels may be used as well as sport drinks, again keeping firmly in mind that fructose is vital, so that glucose uptake into the liver is optimized.

There is one physiological truth, one unsung secret of exercise physiology that needs to be underscored and preached to every exercising youth or adult, every recreational or professional athlete, every coach and sport physiologist. It is this:

Glucokinase must be unlocked from the liver cell and available to allow for glucose uptake by the liver during exercise. Exercise inhibits glucokinase release, but fructose will release this enzyme. Fueling during exercise with fructose and glucose in a balanced ratio facilitates glucose uptake into the liver and promotes glycogen formation. The result is improved power output, improved mental acuity, improved psychology and improved recovery. And with improved recovery comes the added bonus of improved overall health.

After Exercise

There are some important considerations to keep in mind in the post-exercise period. The key is to refuel as quickly as possible after exercise. This not only optimizes replenishment of fuel stores, in particular muscle glycogen, but also readies the body for optimum recovery physiology. Many coaches and trainers will recommend a protein supplement immediately after exercise, and this is perfectly in order. In the immediate post-exercise period usually lasting about 2 hours, uptake of protein is optimized. It makes good sense to take advantage of this. Also the replenishment of muscle glycogen is improved when carbohydrates are ingested during this period along with protein.

The post-exercise replenishment of muscle glycogen may also be achieved with carbohydrate drinks or food. Suitable foods are whole grain breads, pasta, rice and potatoes. These carbs are rapidly metabolized to glucose and are optimal for muscle replenishment in the post-exercise metabolic environment.

During exercise, contracting muscles extract glucose from the circulation with great efficiency. This may seem contradictory because insulin is suppressed during exercise and muscle cells normally require insulin signaling to promote this uptake. Contracting muscles, however, extract glucose from the circulation by a system that is independent of insulin known as exercise-induced muscle uptake of glucose. As each muscle cell contracts, the glucose transporters are driven to the cell wall allowing for rapid glucose uptake, a process normally requiring insulin.

This system, independent of and complementary to insulin, remains in place for up to 48 hours in the post-exercise period and this ensures good muscle glycogen replenishment. Muscle cells will extract up to 90% of available glucose during this period. In addition to this exercise-induced mechanism, insulin will also be released in response to carbohydrate intake, and this will be additive to the exercise induced mechanism.

The post-exercise refueling period must also give attention to replenishing the liver glycogen stores. This will occur if one includes some fructose-containing foods, such as fruits and vegetables or honey, which ensure liver uptake of glucose. Any liver glycogen formed will be quickly released from the liver in this period to provide glucose for depleted muscle tissue as referred to above. Therefore, it is also recommended to do some selective refueling of the liver in the post-exercise period before bedtime when recovery physiology is the key metabolic consideration.

Chapter 7

The Payoff from Proper Brain Fueling

*T*here are three basic metabolic benefits that come from taking care of your brain's energy demands first. They are:

1. Stabilization and control of blood glucose
2. Improved sleep
3. Elimination or reduction of metabolic stress

These benefits are the result of dietary habits that keep the liver glycogen reserve maintained at all times providing energy for the brain when and how it needs it. All three are interrelated. All three are the result of a "simple and inexpensive strategy that involves myth-defying choices" such as eating something before bedtime.[57]

Following nutritional guidelines based on the Glycemic Index or adhering to a well-intended but misguided focus on carbohydrates or calorie counting will not automatically produce these benefits. They are derived only as the result of an intentional strategy that begins and ends with liver glycogen formation, a strategy never mentioned in nutritional counseling or dietary advice given to diabetics or those suffering from sleep disorders or any of the other conditions related to the metabolic syndrome. Here are the facts.

Stabilization and Control of Blood Sugar

First, an adequate liver glycogen reserve means that blood sugar levels are stabilized and controlled. When blood sugar is low as during exercise or sleep, liver glycogen will be released to fuel the brain and the muscles if needed. When blood sugar is low as in reactive hypoglycemia or other forms of hypoglycemia, liver glycogen is released to increase the blood sugar level.

The ingestion of foods that form liver glycogen directly (those containing fructose and glucose in nearly equal ratios) allows for glucose to be brought into the liver to form liver glycogen. Thus, blood glucose levels do not rise as much as would be expected when consuming an equal amount of starchy foods. When blood glucose is stable and liver glycogen levels are replete, the brain is guaranteed a continuous supply of fuel.

Improved Sleep

Second, when liver glycogen levels are maintained at optimal levels, the brain's energy needs during rest is ensured. Sleep patterns improve. Recovery sleep occurs uninterrupted throughout the night. The brain, which functions in a high energy state during rest, can count on an adequate fuel supply and will not initiate actions designed to procure fuel for itself during sleep.

Proper brain fueling before bedtime not only improves sleep patterns but also results in numerous health benefits that are the direct result of improved sleep. These range from reductions in the risks for hypertension and cardiovascular disease to improved learning and memory.

Elimination or Reduction of Metabolic Stress

Third, when the brain is well fueled throughout the day and at night during sleep, it has no need to initiate metabolic stress. Metabolic stress, often referred to as the "fight or flight" response, is a protective mechanism initiated at times when the brain senses that its fuel supply is inadequate or running low. Cortisol and adrenalin are released from the adrenal glands to stimulate the release of glycogen from the liver and keep glucose in the blood circulation for use by the brain.

Elimination or reduction of recurrent metabolic stress is the most significant beneficial result of a well-fueled brain. The well-known risks for many conditions and diseases that are the result of chronic and repeated metabolic stress can be greatly reduced or eliminated altogether.

We will get to these in more detail in the next chapter. For now we want to focus on prevention and the benefits that can be derived from meeting your brain's energy needs.

"The problem with prevention is that it requires a disciplined practice of delayed gratification."

Prevention must begin early. Children as young as 10 to 12 years old are increasingly being diagnosed with Type 2 (adult-onset) diabetes. Nearly 20% of teenagers are obese. 65% our total population is overweight or obese. Alzheimer's disease, unheard of in the 1950s and 1960s, now affects one in four families. Sleep disorders are epidemic. Depression, ADHD, cognitive learning deficits, osteoporosis, hypothyroidism and dementia drive pharmaceutical solutions to the tune of billions of dollars annually.

The problem with *prevention* is that it requires a disciplined practice of delayed gratification. We cannot immediately see or may never see the results. It is difficult to appreciate the full effect of choices that could have eliminated many of these conditions and diseases.

Instead, our tendency is to focus on the short term, the fad diet, the quick fix, and the pill that promises to lower our numbers. We spend billions of dollars on drugs that give us a tangible sense of doing something. Our numbers (blood glucose, cholesterol, etc.) do come down, but the reality is, the underlying condition (chronic brain starvation resulting in chronic metabolic stress) may not be affected at all.

"We have become so exercised in pursuing minutia ("straining out gnats") in our dietary recommendations that we sometimes lose sight of the mountain of damage we heap on ourselves daily by the excessive consumption of sugars and HFCS ("swallowing camels").

Another widespread practice of contemporary society is to accept the claims of selected, heavily marketed yet narrowly targeted food supplements and additives with their pseudo-scientific health claims. We are led to believe that oatmeal and Cheerios are heart healthy and cholesterol lowering, and that low-fat yogurt is better for you. We swallow fish oil and CoQ10 capsules and probiotics, all in the hopes of preventing some feared medical outcome. We indulge in cleansings and purges to rid ourselves of toxins that we believe will harm us, and which, by the way, our body does a pretty good job of eliminating naturally.

All the while, our brains are starving and initiating metabolic conditions that really do kill us and deprive us of health. Our over indulgent diets are filled with sugars and carbohydrates and HFCS, which result in insulin resistance and ultimately in the metabolic syndrome and all of its associated conditions and diseases. It all reminds me of an analogy that Jesus used in the New Testament when criticizing the hypocrisy exhibited by the teachers of the Law. "You blind guides!" he said. "You strain out a gnat but swallow a camel."[58]

When it comes to experts in nutrition, and many of our medical professionals, we are "blind guides." We have become so exercised in pursuing minutia ("straining out gnats") in our dietary recommendations that we sometimes lose sight of the mountain of damage we heap on ourselves daily by the excessive consumption of sugars and HFCS ("swallowing camels").

Eric's Story

*E*ric was lying beside the mountain path at 8,300 feet elevation when the search and rescue team found him. He had gone for a hike that morning and was making his descent when he felt a sharp stabbing pain in his left shoulder. He had a hard time catching his breath, rested for a moment and tried to continue downward to the trailhead where his car was parked. When the pain resumed with what seemed to be constricting pressure over his mid chest area, he had clarity enough to abandon his descent, call 911 on his cell phone, give his location and wait for help.

Eric was 69. In earlier years he was a marathon runner (he had completed over 30 marathons) and in midlife had taken up mountain biking and hiking. He was not overweight, but closer inspection revealed a midsection flabbiness that seemed inconsistent with his muscular legs and trim upper body. He had no history of heart disease.

The cardiac monitor in the ambulance on the way to the emergency room showed acute and dramatic changes. Fortunately for Eric, he reached the hospital, was immediately admitted to the electro-physiology cardiac lab. Three stints were placed in one coronary artery which was effectively 100% occluded, and another stint was placed in another artery that showed 70% occlusion. Eric survived, but questions lingered.

Eric's story reminds one of the first-person commercials you see on TV for Bayer aspirin. The couple is sitting on the couch and the very fit-looking husband says, "I was in perfect health and out of the blue I had a heart attack." How can one explain coronary artery occlusion (heart attack) in an otherwise seasoned runner and avid exerciser in supposedly perfect health? The answer is predictable though not widely understood within a context of conventional wisdom.

There can be only one explanation, which also informs us why over 50% of those suffering heart attacks have normal cholesterol measurements. For many, fats, or being fat, are not the problem underlying the acute onset of heart disease like Eric experienced. Metabolic stress, underscored by chronic or repeated release of elevated levels of cortisol and adrenalin due to brain starvation (the hallmark of the metabolic syndrome) is the problem.

That indeed was Eric's problem. Here is how it began. Eric was a brilliant mathematician and academician. He taught at a prestigious military academy. He was driven in his pursuit of excellence in his teaching and personal life, which meant he was early to work, late to leave, frequently skipped meals, especially breakfast, snacked on junk food and consumed large amounts of coffee throughout the day and then wound down by taking long runs or bike rides without proper fueling before or after.

He didn't sleep well and frequently awakened between 3:00 and 4:00 AM unable to get back to sleep for 45 minutes to an hour, only to be awakened by his alarm at 5:30 AM so that he could arrive for work before 7:30 AM. Breakfast, if he took the time to gulp it down, consisted of cereal or toast and coffee. Once at work, the coffee was free and donuts and pastries were readily available throughout the morning and that seemed to keep him going. Lunch, when he could take time for it, was hurried and overloaded with starch or carbohydrates which shot his blood sugar up only to be followed by excessive insulin release and a subsequent rapidly falling blood glucose leaving him hungry again by mid afternoon. Again, coffee and snacks filled in temporarily until supper.

He seldom ate fruit, but consumed large amounts of vegetables in season that he grew in his garden. He didn't eat much red meat, avoided fatty foods, and consumed low-fat options when he could. He avoided any food before bedtime that he believed would only be unnecessary energy during sleep and would only turn to fat. He assumed his diet was heart healthy never once considering that his diet was at the heart of his heart problem.

Eric was experiencing metabolic stress for more than 18 to 20 hours of every day. His brain was silently monitoring its fuel reserve in the liver and found it wanting. From nearly 10:00 PM every evening until shortly after lunch, no liver glycogen was available directly from food intake. The brain had no recourse but to manufacture it from amino acids available from muscle protein. His long periods of exercise, experienced three to five times a week were undertaken with depleted liver glycogen stores, further driving metabolic stress and muscle protein cannibalism just to fuel his hungry brain.

When he did eat, his carbohydrate consumption succeeded in raising his blood sugar temporarily, only to be followed by an excessive release of insulin that in 90 to 120 minutes left him with little liver glycogen produced and little to no liver glycogen to fuel his brain during the night.

Fortunately, good genetics had protected Eric from obesity and early onset of diabetes, and other conditions and diseases on the metabolic stress continuum. But good genes could not protect Eric from decades of metabolic stress directed at his cardiovascular system, and on approaching the beginning of his eighth decade of life, it finally caught up with him.

The good news is that Eric's heart attack did not end his life. He was given a reprieve. A change in diet, which included proper fueling before and after exercise, and before bedtime promised to give Eric many more productive years of computational instruction and good health.

Chapter 8

Fast Track

- The immediate consequence of failure to fuel the brain properly is metabolic (adrenal-driven) stress.
- Continued, repeated metabolic stress over time may result in some or all of the conditions and diseases known as the metabolic syndrome.
- The hormonal cascade that begins with low liver glycogen levels and leads to the conditions and diseases of the metabolic syndrome can be prevented.

The Consequences of Failure to Fuel the Brain Properly

*T*he consequences of failure to fuel the brain properly can be viewed as a continuum that begins with the immediate or short-term consequences and progresses ultimately over time to involve longer-term risks. Throughout the book so far, we have noted that the most immediate effect of inadequate brain fueling is metabolic stress triggered by an increase in IGFBP-1 produced in the liver in response to low liver glycogen levels.

Metabolic stress is a specialized from of stress mediated by the brain affecting almost every organ of our bodies. Metabolic stress is something we do to ourselves. We can't blame it on genetics, although the ultimate result of metabolic stress or the degree to which one is affected by stress may be determined by our genes. It may be triggered by external environmental or social factors or by internal emotions, but its primary cause is failure to properly provide cerebral energy.

Metabolic stress is the direct result of poor choices that we make, typically involving lifestyle, food, and nutrition. It is real. It is not accidental. It is internal. It happens. Most of us experience metabolic stress from time to time and over 25% of us have medical conditions associated with it. The prevalence of these conditions increases with age. The key organs involved in short-term metabolic stress are the liver and the brain. Long-term consequences involve nearly every organ in the body.

The Metabolic Stress Continuum

If we were to picture the conditions related to metabolic stress as a continuum shown in the inverted triangle that follows, metabolic stress would occupy the position at the lower portion of the inverted triangle. Above metabolic stress, in ascending order of significance, would be all the conditions associated with glucose intolerance, including insulin resistance, weight gain and elevations in triglycerides and other lipids. Above insulin resistance is the metabolic syndrome,

Type 2 diabetes, hypertension, and serum cholesterol and triglyceride elevations. Finally, a host of other chronic inflammatory diseases associated with age and diabetes including cardiovascular disease, hypertension, thyroid diseases, and neuro-degenerative conditions including Alzheimer's disease, various forms of dementia and Parkinsonism.

The Metabolic Stress Continuum

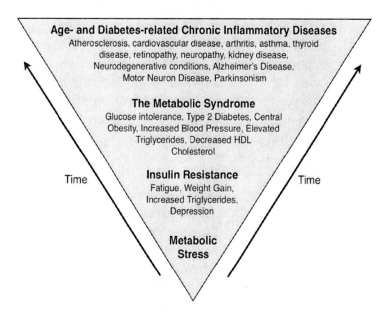

Describing the symptoms and conditions in this way is not meant to communicate that the levels or categories indicated by this progression are distinct. Rather, the "boundaries" between the levels are overlapping as one ascends from the bottom to the top. All the conditions and diseases, however, are linked to a common metabolic cause. Furthermore, viewing metabolic stress as a continuum is not meant to imply that the conditions or diseases are progressive in a linear sense, that is, one must first experience a clinical condition or disease on a lower level of the diagram before one contracts a clinical condition or disease on a level above, though such may be the case. It must be pointed out again that one's genetic code and lifestyle may play a significant role in determining the extent to which one is possibly afflicted by the conditions and diseases of this metabolic stress continuum.

When viewing the continuum from a therapeutic or clinical point of view, it is interesting to observe that treatment interventions are usually begun at the upper levels of the triangle rather than at the lower "causative" level. Yet interventions begun at the level of causation (metabolic stress) may be more effective in terms of limiting morbidity or preventing the progression of future conditions or diseases.

Metabolic stress is internal physiologic stress. It happens as the result of activation of a cascade of stress hormones from the hypothalamus, the pituitary and adrenal glands (the hypothalmus-pituitary-adrenal or HPA axis). The action of the HPA axis triggers the release of adrenal stress hormones also known as glucocorticoids. These hormones are adrenalin and cortisol, sometimes referred to as "fight or flight" hormones, but they should be more correctly referred to as neuroprotective hormones for their essential purpose is to ensure that the brain has adequate fuel for functioning at all times, especially during times of physical stress.

The brain must depend on fuel, primarily glucose, delivered by the circulating blood for its energy supply. On its own, the brain would run out of energy necessary to function properly in about 30 seconds. It is because of this very small fuel reserve that the "fight or flight"

HPA reflex is so important to survival. Here we refer to this reflex as neuro-protective, for without it the brain would quickly lapse into coma and cease functioning.

Only glycogen from the liver storehouse is available for other organs and tissues in the body. Though the glycogen storage capacity of skeletal muscle is more than ten times that of the liver, muscle glycogen is not shared. Once glucose enters the muscle cell and forms glycogen, it stays there and is not available for use by the rest of the body. This fact is often lost on those who consider total glycogen storage capacity (liver and skeletal muscle glycogen) as a single fuel source for metabolic needs of the body.

The "Stress Hormone Cascade" shown on page 134 summarizes the metabolic events leading up to the metabolic syndrome. In addition to the specific conditions and diseases of the metabolic syndrome as currently defined, we can also include many sleep disorders, hypothyroid conditions, and neuro-degenerative diseases in this progression of conditons whose etiology begins with failure to provide the brain with adequate fuel from the liver glycogen reserve.

The duration, severity, and frequency of occurence of episodes of metabolic stress would also seem to play a role in the development of the conditions and diseases along this continuum. For some, it may take decades for disease to manifest itself. For others, only months or years. It seems that the body responds more negatively to multiple repeated insults than it may to one chronic exposure. In other words, repeated failure to fuel the brain resulting in metabolic stress night after night and associated sleep loss may have a more significant negative effect on health than a single episode of starvation or stress from a bout of an infectious disease.

The Stress Hormone Cascade

FROM LOW LIVER GLYCOGEN LEVELS TO THE METABOLIC SYNDROME

- **LOW LIVER GLYCOGEN** levels trigger the release of
  - Elevated levels of IGFBP-1 which are associated with
    - Elevated levels of the 11beta-HSD-1 which
      - Activate intracellular cortisone producing
        - Increased metabolic stress which results in
          - Conditions and diseases known as

THE METABOLIC SYNDROME

Which includes the following:

- Insulin resistance, fasting hyperglycemia, Type 2 diabetes mellitus or impaired fasting glucose, impaired glucose tolerance
- Hypertension or elevated blood pressure
- Central obesity (also known as visceral, male-pattern or apple-shaped adiposity), overweight with fat deposits mainly around the waist
- Decreased HDL cholesterol (a risk for heart disease)
- Elevated triglycerides and other associated diseases

We do know that it only takes a few days of sleep deprivation to produce a dramatic change in one's metabolic profile. In 1999, Professor Van Cauter and her team at Chicago University found that a loss of four hours of sleep each night for only six nights in otherwise healthy young men resulted in alteration of their metabolic profile from that of a healthful state to that consistent with obesity and Type 2 diabetes. This is an astonishing reversal of a healthy profile in such a short period of time. It serves to reinforce the message warning of the devastating consequences of this form of metabolism experienced by many over months, years and even decades.

The metabolic stress continuum is interrelated with two additional closely related factors. One way of describing this interwoven relationship is as a toxic three-stranded metabolic cord comprised of the dual strands of *chronic partial nocturnal brain starvation* and *chronic partial sleep loss*, which synergistically activate the third strand of *chronic metabolic stress* mediated by the HPA axis. These three strands are so tightly inter-related as to make them virtually inseparable. The binding and destructive effects of this toxic cord impact every organ system and metabolic function in the body, eventually resulting in the conditions and diseases that are collectively known as the metabolic syndrome.

It is the chronic repeated partial starvation of the brain from inadequate liver glycogen levels night after night, year after year that drives this metabolic stress continuum, contributing to sleep loss and the initiation of a profound metabolic response over time. The list of the conditions produced by this "toxic cord" is long and includes: [59]

- Obesity
- Diabetes
- Heart disease
- High blood pressure
- Hyperlipidemia (elevated cholesterol and triglycerides)
- Some forms of cancer
- Osteoporosis
- Polycystic ovarian disease
- Sleep disorders including insomnia, sleep apnea
- Dementia
- Neuro-degenerative diseases including Alzheimer's Disease, Parkinsonism, and motor neuron disease (Lou Gehrig's disease)
- Depression
- Immune system compromise
- Hypothyroidism
- Arthritis
- Kidney disease
- Chronic fatigue
- Menopausal symptoms
- Infertility
- Gastrointestinal diseases
- ADHD (attention deficit hyperactivity disorder)

Elizabeth's Story

*E*lizabeth was in her early sixties when her husband began noticing changes. Car keys would "disappear." The burner on the stove would be left on after meal preparation was complete. Words would be missed in casual conversation – everyday words with well-known meanings seemed to be forgotten. Her dress habits, which had always been proper, even immaculate at times, seemed to slip occasionally – the same outfit two days in a row or jewelry that didn't quite match or confusion about what went with what. At times, she just appeared "lost" or lonely and withdrawn.

It all happened so subtly without fanfare or warning. It "just wasn't like her" was the way her husband described her mental state to her physician. Physical examination and multiple diagnostic tests revealed that Elizabeth was experiencing the early onset of Alzheimer's disease (AD). Except for having adult-onset diabetes for several years, Elizabeth was, by her family's admission, in fairly good health. She had no history of high blood pressure or strokes or heart irregularities. Her memory, until recent months, had been exceptional. Everyone who knew her considered her bright and outgoing. No one in her family had experienced anything like this, no dementia, no strokes, no premature memory loss.

"How could this be happening?" her husband questioned. Their lives were happy and uncomplicated. Their interests centered on family, which lived close, and several grandchildren who Elizabeth doted on with regularity. Now, even the youngest wondered at times if Grandma was all right.

Virtually unheard of before the sixties, Alzheimer's disease now touches nearly one in five extended families and by 2050 is projected to affect one in 85 individuals worldwide. Its increase in incidence has been attributed to many factors, though no specific causative factors have been isolated. Individuals with hypertension, increased cholesterol, diabetes, and a history of smoking seem to have a higher risk for developing AD.

For Elizabeth and her family, the thought of experiencing a tortuous march toward certain mental deterioration with little hope for treatment seemed devastating.

What clues exist that might lead to an understanding of Elizabeth's plight? The discoveries of medical science over the past 40 years give us few to consider. But by connecting the dots linking Elizabeth's metabolic history, some general insights are possible.

The chronic elevation in blood sugar (hyperglycemia) that characterized Elizabeth's diabetes produced a chronic elevation in insulin release (hyperinsulinemia) that eventually resulted in insulin resistance, a condition where the insulin that is produced is not effective. From the brain's perspective, this deprives the individual brain cells (neurons) of needed energy by a process known as increased intracellular oxidative stress. Over time, the brain cells ability to generate ATP (the energy source within the mitochondria of each neuron) is decreased or compromised. When the mitochondria fail, glucose cannot be absorbed into the glial cells of the brain, those cells responsible for delivering the fuel supply to each neuron. Without energy, brain cells cannot function properly and eventually die.

At the same time, another sinister action takes place within the synapses (the interspaces between neurons) of the brain. Glutamate, the primary brain signal neuro-transmitter, accumulates within the synapses due to the failure of the mitochondria to generate ATP properly. This accumulation of glutamate is toxic to brain tissue, further compromising brain function and resulting in chronic levels of cortisol to be released from the adrenal glands.

Increased cortisol levels have a profoundly negative effect on the hippocampus, the portion of the brain most responsible for memory consolidation, short-term memory and learning, contributing to the loss of recent memory. [See Appendix D for a flow diagram that summarizes these complex metabolic challenges.]

While one cannot be entirely certain that this catastrophic chain of events was responsible for Elizabeth's AD, the logic points in that direction. Over the years, she consumed more and more carbohydrates, partly in an attempt to "eat healthy" by cutting down on fat. Decades of high carbohydrate consumption (especially simple sugars) resulted in chronically elevated blood sugar levels that led to insulin resistance, diabetes and ultimately to the loss of brain function that resulted in her early symptoms of AD.[60]

Chapter 9

> **Fast Track**
>
> - The dietary strategy presented here emphasizes fueling your brain first rather than a focus on calorie counting or carbohydrate consumption.
> - This brain-first strategy is a much more sensible approach to eating.
> - Gram-for-gram, honey is the highest-octane brain fuel, resulting in the greatest liver glycogen yield.
> - The principles of the "brain-first dietary revolution" will keep your brain happy and well fueled.
> - Proper food intake to replenish liver glycogen reserves in a timely fashion should be matched with times the brain is most at risk of fuel shortage.
> - The target Liver Glycogen Yield for every meal or snack should be about 75 grams.
> - Ten grams of liver glycogen will fuel the brain for about one hour at rest.

*B*rowse in any large bookstore and one can choose from hundreds of cookbooks, recipe books and diet books that fill the shelves. Even your local grocer now sells dozens of cookbooks and menu planners. Peal back the label of many processed foods and underneath will be recipes and serving options. Browse the internet for diets and one would not live long enough to read them all. The selections are overwhelming.

One of the definitions of "revolution" is "a fundamental change in the way of thinking about or visualizing something: a change of paradigm . . ."[61] The purpose in writing this book is to get you to abandon the dietary strategies that focus primarily on control of blood sugar (e.g., the glycemic index based diets and others that seem to have a calorie or carbohydrate fetish) and the elimination of saturated fats. After all, it was the "avoid saturated fats" and "low-fat" craze that started in the 70s and 80s that got us into the fat epidemic that we see all around us. Every cattle farmer knows that the best way to fatten up cattle for market is feed them corn, a vegetable made up of over 70% starch or glucose.[62] That's exactly what the dietary emphasis on low-fat foods has wrought, a generation of folks who have been fattened up with carbohydrates, especially HFCS made from cornstarch! [63]

Medical science and practice for the past several decades has been fixated, it seems, on blood glucose concentration. The goal of treatment for blood glucose abnormalities has been to "control the numbers" with a combination of medicines. But blood glucose is not an accurate measure of the body's total glucose control. In other words, blood glucose does not tell us anything about the body's energy homeostasis (or balance) at any given moment. It is not an index or measure of underlying metabolic "weather" nor an indicator of underlying metabolic conditions. Most certainly, blood glucose measurement does not tell us anything about the most vital metabolic index of all, the liver glycogen status - the only true index of ongoing energy provision for the brain.

Earlier we have seen that any derivative measure or index related to blood glucose is shortsighted and incomplete. While it is impressive to consider the International Table of Glycemic Index and Load (reproduced in part in Appendix C) and the calculated values for hundreds of foods that have been tested, we would simply point out again that any measure or indicator based on blood glucose concentration is transient and essentially meaningless with regard to liver glycogen formation and brain fuel reserve.

Though blood glucose (and the related glucose tolerance test or GTT) has been relied on for decades as an indicator of blood glucose control and treatment recommendations, these provide only a temporary and frequently misleading indication of the brain's fuel status and fuel availability. Even the HbA1c (glycohemoglobin) test used today as a more reliable indicator of average blood glucose over several weeks cannot provide information on liver glycogen status or brain fuel availability.

A more important and nutritionally relevant measure would be one that indicates a food's ability to form liver glycogen, the fuel reserve for the brain. That measure, introduced in Chapter 5, is the *brain fuel indicator* (BFI) or IGFBP-1.

It may be revolutionary, but paying attention to the energy requirements of the brain in the selection of the foods that we eat and the timing of when we eat them is important. This idea may not be intuitive for you at first. We have all grown up with the idea that three meals a day is right and proper. And eating before bedtime is to be avoided. Yet, concern for meeting the energy requirements of the brain drives us to consider different eating habits than those with which we may be accustomed or familiar.

"A much more sensible approach to eating, yet one that is 'undiscovered' in a practical sense is to consider a dietary strategy that considers the fuel requirements of the brain first, at every meal or snack time."

Honey is High Octane Brain Fuel

Think of it as a fueling strategy for providing your body with a "high-octane" fuel. Just as higher-octane fuel in your car will give a high-performance engine a boost in horsepower, so will consuming a high-octane food in a timely manner provide your brain with a consistent supply of quality energy.

Gram for gram, honey is the highest-octane food you can consume, for it results in the greatest yield of liver glycogen. Yield in this case is not measured by the total calories or carbohydrates consumed. Nor is yield primarily concerned with blood glucose levels such as is the focus of the glycemic index and diets based on it.

A much more sensible approach to nutrition, yet one that is "undiscovered" in a practical sense, is to consider a dietary strategy that considers the fuel requirements of the brain first. In the following chapters, we will give you a few practical suggestions about meals, snacks and an over-all nutritional plan. We have even included several brain-healthy recipes including foods that promote liver glycogen formation.

First, let's summarize a few basic principles of a new "brain-first" dietary revolution that will keep your brain happy.

Principles of the "Brain-first" Dietary Revolution

1. It is better to eat multiple times a day – five times a day or more if your exercise level demands it – but eat less at each meal (we'll tell you how much later). Eating two or three times a day is not "brain smart."

2. Choose foods that fuel your brain, that is, foods that result in a higher yield of liver glycogen formation directly at every meal or snack.

3. Remember the liver glycogen reserve is quite small. Don't exceed its storage capacity or the liver's ability to metabolize sugar by consuming foods or drinks that overwhelm it with excessive fructose at any meal or snack.

4. Be less concerned about fats and more concerned about excessive consumption of sugar and HFCS. Eliminate excessive sugar and HFCS from your diet. Remember, you do not get fat by eating fat. You get fat by consuming too much sugar and HFCS.

5. Avoid skipping meals or going on short term fasts as a way of losing weight. You only trigger repeated cycles of metabolic stress that result in more fat storage when you resume eating.

6. Stay away from artificial sweeteners. The sweet taste sensors on the tongue alert the brain. The brain thinks that a sweet, calorie rich food is incoming and alerts the insulin producing cells in the pancreas which then release more insulin. Insulin drives circulating glucose out of the blood into the cells and out of reach of the hungry brain. The blood sugar drops, triggering a release of appetite stimulating hormones and

another round of metabolic stress. Studies show that most who use artificial sweeteners regularly end up gaining weight.

When to Eat and Why

In Chapter 6, we described in detail the times of the day when the brain is potentially at risk from fuel shortages. Matching those high-risk times with proper food intake designed to replenish liver glycogen reserves and fuel the brain is a great starting place in this revolutionary nutritional strategy.

Breakfast. Most dietary experts will tell you that breakfast is the most important meal of the day. But few will be able to tell you the number one reason why that is true. On awakening, liver glycogen levels will be at their lowest, even lower than after an hour or so of intense exercise. It is important that the first meal of the day includes foods that will result in the rapid and direct formation of liver glycogen.

Here is where the logic of depending on blood glucose measurements begins to fall apart. As we have noted, blood sugar may be elevated on awakening even though no food has been consumed since the early evening of the day before, more than 12 hours or more in some cases. If one bases food intake on the fact that blood sugar is already elevated, one would be tempted to avoid eating at all. On the other hand, if blood sugar was low, one may be tempted to consume carbohydrates that rapidly raise blood sugar. Both strategies would be shortsighted and have adverse health consequences in the near term. When repeated day after day, for months or years, the negative health consequences are multiplied.

Midmorning. If your first meal of the day was early, 6:00 to 7:00 AM, your liver glycogen levels will be nearly depleted by noon. Rather than wait until IGFBP-1, the brain fuel indicator, begins to be released from the liver as an early warning sign, why not prevent an unnecessary initiation of metabolic stress by having a midmorning snack of foods containing a balance of fructose and glucose needed to restock liver glycogen.

Lunch. By noontime, the liver glycogen store will again be nearly depleted (assuming you have had a good breakfast including some protein, fruit and honey). It is time to replenish the tank for the long afternoon haul. Lunch is the meal that provides almost infinite flexibility and fits every particular nutritional predilection from vegetarian to bring-on-the-beef.

Again, the emphasis should be on maximizing the liver glycogen (brain fuel) store. For most, it may be six or seven hours until dinner. Even sedentary activities or light work during the afternoon requires the release of at least ten grams per hour of liver glycogen to fuel the brain, kidneys and red blood cells. By dinner the fuel reserve for the brain will be just about depleted.

Late Afternoon. As with the midmorning snack, a midafternoon snack can ensure that the brain has enough fuel to make it through to dinnertime.

Dinner. Whether you are utilitarian in your meal preparation or love to cook, dinner is the time for creativity and imagination. But as with every other meal or snack, be sure to include fruits with their balance of fructose and glucose, some vegetables and protein which is broken down to amino acids, also necessary in liver glycogen formation.

147

Bedtime. Next to breakfast, a bedtime refueling stop is the most important of the day. What you eat at bedtime is critical and must be focused on rapidly replenishing the liver glycogen reserve, topping it off just before rest.

What you eat and how much you consume is somewhat dependent on the time that you had dinner and what you may have been doing since that last meal of the day. If dinner included proteins, fruit and vegetables, the liver would have been busy forming liver glycogen from the fructose and glucose obtained from fruits, and from amino acids from proteins. By 10:00 or 11:00 PM the liver glycogen reserve may be nearly full (75 grams).

If, however, dinner consisted mainly of carbohydrates, which comprise the bulk of most American meals (typically up to 80% carbohydrates for many), blood sugar would have spiked about 8:00 PM and the increased insulin release would have driven blood sugar into muscle and fat cells so that by bedtime, blood sugar would be falling. Liver glycogen would be released to make up for lower blood sugar, leaving less than a full reserve tank for brain fuel during the night.

Consuming fruits at bedtime may force the digestive tract to stay "awake" digesting fiber and pulp. Excess water from juices may not be the best just before bed either. That is why honey is the gold-standard food to consume before sleep. It is quickly digested and forms liver glycogen directly in the liver. And honey promotes sleep via the HYMN cycle.[64]

How Much Is Too Much?

The goal of this brain-first dietary strategy is to eat properly in order to avoid running out of brain fuel reserves at any time during the 24-hour cycle.

The discerning reader also needs to consider the consequences of *exceeding* the target of keeping the liver glycogen reserve replete. In other words, how much is too much?

The answer lies in knowing the capacity of the tank and understanding how fuel resources are selectively proportioned into the tank. As we have indicated several times, the capacity of the liver glycogen reserve is about 75 grams. For some, the capacity may be up to 110 grams, but 75 grams is understood to be average across all body sizes. Foods that rapidly contribute to the formation of liver glycogen (e.g., foods that contain nearly equal proportions of fructose and glucose) include fruits, some vegetables and honey. That is, consuming these foods will result in liver glycogen formation within 30 to 60 minutes.

In order to fill up the tank, one would need to consume approximately five Tbsp of honey at one time. Any more and the capacity of the tank to form and store glycogen would be exceeded. Excess fructose and glucose would be converted to triglycerides and/or dumped back into the blood where it would be delivered to muscle and fat cells for storage as fat. Of course, eating this much honey at one time is not recommended, especially if it is consumed with other foods. Perhaps this explains the warning given in Proverbs: "If you find honey, eat just enough — too much of it, and you will vomit." (Proverbs 25:16)

A similar statement regarding glycogen formation can be made for fruits. One medium apple contains about the same amount of fructose and glucose as one Tbsp of honey. Therefore the capacity of the liver to form and store the sugars from an apple would be exceeded with the consumption of five apples, probably not an amount that would typically be consumed by anyone.

"Any mixed meal or snack that contains a total of more than 75 grams of fructose and glucose presents the liver with more sugar than it can process and store."

The important principle here is that foods that have an equal balance of fructose and glucose contribute to the rapid formation of liver glycogen. Foods that have an excess amount of sucrose, glucose or starch (foods like potatoes, rice, breads, and cereals as well as some fruits like bananas) do not form liver glycogen as effectively. The high amount of glucose triggers a huge release of insulin from the pancreas. Insulin drives the glucose into the cells where it is stored for energy or converted to fat. Any mixed meal or snack that contains a total of more than 75 grams of fructose and glucose presents the liver with more sugar than it can process and store. This fact underscores why the Liver Glycogen Yield from foods is such an important part of a dietary strategy.

Proteins and the amino acids derived from them are different to a degree. While amino acids can contribute directly to the formation of glycogen in the liver, it takes more time to digest a protein meal and deliver the amino acids to the liver for processing. Therefore, 75 grams of protein, while it may result in the formation of 45 to 50 grams of liver glycogen ultimately, does not have an immediate effect on liver glycogen formation.

Fats do not under any circumstances form sugar or glycogen. Therefore they are not considered relevant in the discussion regarding liver glycogen yield.

One other general principle to remember is that ten grams of liver glycogen will provide fuel for the brain for about one hour at rest. This is especially critical to remember when choosing foods to snack on before bedtime. One should avoid sugary drinks and high carb snacks that simply raise blood sugar (rather than produce glycogen in the liver) and prompt an insulin release leaving little glucose in the blood for the brain after 60 to 90 minutes.

In summary, menu selections or choices for between-meal snacks, should have as a target, a total liver glycogen yield of 70 to 80 grams. When a meal includes proteins, that target may be exceeded by 25 to 50% given the fact that it will take two to three hours or more for the amino acids to reach the liver for conversion into glycogen.

Chapter 10 – Recipes

> **Fast Track**
>
> - This book is intended to be a sampler of recipes and menus that maximize Liver Glycogen Yield (LGY) with every meal or snack.
> - The Liver Glycogen Yield given for each recipe in the chapters that follow may be the most important part of the recipe.
> - Instructions are given when substituting honey for sugar in cooking and baking.

*M*any of you have skipped the first nine chapters and jumped right to the recipes. Congratulations! You, like a majority of folks don't really care why a nutritional strategy does or does not work. You just want to get started. Forget the science or physiology. "Just show me what to eat and how to cook so that I can lose weight and I'm happy."

A few caveats are necessary before the recipes, however. First, this is not intended to be a comprehensive recipe book, but rather a sampler of recipes and menus that show you how to maximize liver glycogen yield with every meal or snack.

There are many wonderful recipe books that feature honey. One of my favorites is *The Buzz on Honey* by Marcella Richman. A few recipes from her collection are included and referenced in the following chapters. If you want more recipes, a quick search for "honey" on www.FoodNetwork.com will result in more than 3000 suggestions in a dozen different categories. Another good source for recipes that use honey is the National Honey Board's website (www.honey.com) recipe section.

One suggestion is to use the recipes in the next few chapters as examples and then look for variations in either of these sites. To that end, I have included recipe names (not complete recipes) found in these two sources and identified where you can find the full recipe. My intent is to expand your list of possibilities. If you want more, just search for "honey recipes" on any search engine and you will find thousands of additional options.

Recipes seem to have a life of their own. They get handed down from generation to generation, scribbled on the back of napkins, or passed on orally at dinner parties. It is not my intent to plagiarize anyone's recipe, and where possible, credit is given to the original source of the recipe. Many of the recipes included herein, however, have no known source. I apologize in advance if a recipe looks just like Aunt Darlene's famous cheesecake or Uncle Harold's Bar-B-Q sauce. I don't even take credit for my own "original" recipes. Someone, somewhere, at sometime has probably made something similar or identical.

If you need detailed step-by-step instructions that begin with "first add two cups of water to a pan, turn on the stove, and heat the water to boiling" this recipe section may not be for you. Cooking, unlike baking (or space flight or brain surgery), is not an exact science. It's OK to experiment and try different things in different combinations and amounts. Generally, being a trial and error kind of a cook, with a lot of informed trial and some errors is acceptable.

What follows are a few specifics and many options. After all, a medical professional is not a clone of Julia Child! I have tried to lend some specificity to the directions for the faint of heart, but for the most part, these recipes will just give you ideas.

The Liver Glycogen Yield "may be the most important part of the recipe."

Where it is possible and appropriate for the food selections used, I have included a calculation of the Liver Glycogen Yield (LGY) that is possible from a particular food or recipe. This may be the most important part of the recipe, as the intent is to maximize this value at each meal or snack time when possible. Some foods, of course, contribute little to liver glycogen formation. They are included to give the reader an indication of the "empty" calories most of us ingest everyday.

Most of the recipes included below use honey. The reason is that honey is the "gold standard" among carbohydrates when it comes to liver glycogen formation. So I include it, even in the cocktail recipes. And when honey is not used in a recipe, you may find it in a sauce or glaze or dressing, just because it adds to the liver glycogen yield.

To give you an idea of just how much liver glycogen is formed from honey compared to other foods, see **Appendix A**. This list attempts to compare the liver glycogen yield on a serving-to-serving basis, with one tablespoon of honey used as a standard serving. Even its closest competitor - dates or raisins - requires nearly 4 times that amount (one quarter cup) to produce as much liver glycogen.

Finally, and most importantly, have fun with cooking. Life is to short to have to cook and/or eat boring food. So enjoy, and remember that when your brain is happy, the whole body is happy!

Substitution of Honey for Sugar

Folks ask frequently, "What about substituting honey for sugar?" The answer depends on whether you are cooking or baking. Here are a few facts to keep in mind. First, some varietals of honey will taste much sweeter than table sugar, some not as sweet. That should only encourage you to try several varietals of honey and use the one that tastes best to you and your family.

Second, when using honey in a recipe, you are adding liquid (honey is ~ 18% water) so it is necessary to reduce the amount of liquid a bit when possible. Third, honey is very acidic. In some recipes, it will be necessary to add baking soda to balance the acidity and to act as a leavening agent. However, if you are adding honey to tomato-based sauces, tomatoes are already acidic and the point is not to neutralize the acid but to balance it with a little sweetness. Also, it is not necessary to add soda when using honey with dairy products - cream, sour cream, yogurt, and cream cheese.

When cooking with honey, or making salad dressings, sauces, marinades, etc., you can simply substitute honey for sugar. You may want to decrease the amount of honey by half and then add more until you arrive at the desired sweetness. In general, one can substitute an amount of honey equal to 2/3 of the amount of sugar called for.

When baking, there are a few suggested rules that you will want to follow if you are using honey. First, you will want to reduce the amount of liquid by ¼ cup for every cup of liquid called for in the recipe. Then you will want to add about ½ teaspoon of baking soda for each cup of honey called for in a recipe. Finally, at lower altitudes, you will want to reduce the oven temperature by 25^0 F, as batters with honey in them tend to brown faster.

Chapter 11 - Appetizers and Snacks

Fruit

*T*here is perhaps nothing better than fresh fruit as a snack midmorning or afternoon or as an appetizer before a meal. All fruit contains nearly equal portions of fructose and glucose, the perfect ratio of these sugars for immediate liver glycogen formation and storage.

Don't save fruit for special occasions or the buffet line. Fruit can be enjoyed everyday, all year in many combinations. Here are some of my favorites for appetizers or snacks that can be eaten raw with all their natural goodness:

Apples - many different varieties (over 10) are available at our grocer year-round. My favorite – Honey Crisp, of course!
Liver Glycogen Yield per serving (1 cup or 1 medium apple): **12 grams**

Grapes - red, green, black
Liver Glycogen Yield per serving (1 cup): **~22 grams**

Oranges - peeled and sliced or wedges
Liver Glycogen Yield per serving (1 cup or 1 orange): ~ **12 grams**

Bananas - great with peanut butter and honey
Liver Glycogen Yield per serving (1 large banana): ~ **15 grams**

Berries - strawberries, raspberries, blackberries, boysenberries, blueberries
Liver Glycogen Yield per serving (1 cup):
Strawberries ~ 7 grams
Raspberries ~ 5 grams
Blackberries ~ 6.5 grams
Boysenberries ~ 8 grams
Blueberries ~ 14 grams

Cherries
Liver Glycogen Yield per serving (1 cup): ~ **20 grams**

Pears
Liver Glycogen Yield per serving (1 cup or 1 pear): ~ **14 grams**

Mellon - watermelon, casaba, honey dew, cantaloupe
Liver Glycogen Yield per serving (1 cup):
Watermelon ~ 8 grams
Casaba ~ 10 grams
Honeydew ~ 12 grams
Cantaloupe ~ 15 grams

Peaches and nectarines
Liver Glycogen Yield per serving (1 cup):
Peaches ~ 11 grams
Nectarines ~ 13 grams

Pineapple
Liver Glycogen Yield per serving (1 cup): ~18 grams

Mangos
Liver Glycogen Yield per serving (1 cup): ~ 20 grams

Papaya
Liver Glycogen Yield per serving (1 cup): ~ 9 grams

Dates
Liver Glycogen Yield per serving (¼ cup): ~ 22 grams

Raisins
Liver Glycogen Yield per serving (¼ cup): ~ 24 grams

Dates and raisins are exceptionally high in fructose and glucose content and both have very little additional sucrose. Raisins also contain amino acids that contribute to the LGY. The approximate liver glycogen yield from seedless raisins (either golden or dark) is over 22 grams per ¼ cup, making them the highest liver glycogen producer of any fruit next to honey.

On average, a serving of fruit will provide 10 to 12 grams of liver glycogen. By adding 2 tablespoons of yogurt and honey dip to the fruit consumed, one can store 16 to 18 grams of glycogen in the liver - that's one-fifth of the total liver glycogen storage capacity from each fruit snack between meals. That's enough for about 2 hours of brain fuel if nothing else is consumed, at least enough to get one to the next meal.

Dips and Dressings to Use with Fruit

Yogurt and honey dip or sauce for fruit

Mix one-cup yogurt (use Greek yogurt if you prefer) with 2 Tbsp of honey. Add a few finely chopped mint leaves, a Tbsp of mint pepper jelly, a teaspoon of chopped candied ginger, a teaspoon of curry powder or ginger, or a Tbsp of finely chopped nuts for variations. Serve over a mixture of fruit or let family or guests choose their fruit favorites from several cut up or sliced selections and add their own topping.

Liver Glycogen Yield per serving (2 Tbsp): ~6 grams

Cream cheese, Parmesan cheese and honey dip

Soften 1 package (8 ounces) of cream cheese (at room temperature). Add 2 Tbsp of Parmesan cheese, two Tbsp of honey and blend thoroughly. For a thinner dip, add a little cream or half and half. For variety, add finely chopped green onions, red bell peppers, roasted red peppers, sun-dried tomatoes or cucumbers.

Liver Glycogen Yield per serving (2 Tbsp): ~6 grams

Honey and curry vegetable dip

This favorite can be made with sour cream, yogurt, cream cheese, mayonnaise or a combination of your choice. If using it as a dip, cream cheese and mayo may work best. Start with one cup of your choice and add 2 Tablespoons of honey. Add 1 teaspoon of curry powder and one or more of the following: raisins, finely chopped vegetables - green, yellow or red bell peppers, roasted red peppers, green onions, cucumbers, radishes, celery, or sweet pickles (about 2 Tbsp total). Mix well and serve with a choice of vegetables.

Liver Glycogen Yield per serving (2 Tbsp): ~ **8 grams** [You can boost the LGY up to **30 grams per serving** if you add chopped raisins or dates.]

Peanut butter and honey (This is not just for kids!)

Mix ½ cup peanut butter (any style but preferably natural peanut butter without added sugar or corn syrup) with 1 to 2 Tbsp of honey. Use as a dip for veggies - carrots, celery, radishes, red or yellow bell peppers.

Liver Glycogen Yield per serving (2 Tbsp): ~ **6 grams**

Honey Lime Sour Cream Dressing[65]

Combine ½ cup sour cream with 3 Tbsp honey and 2 Tbsp lime juice. Serve immediately over cup of combined fruit such as watermelon and honeydew balls with blueberries.

Liver Glycogen Yield per serving (2 Tbsp): ~ **5.7 grams**

Honey Tip: remember that honey is extremely hygroscopic, meaning that it absorbs water. If you use a honey dip or dressing on fruit and mix it ahead of serving time, it will absorb water from the fruit and dilute the dressing.

Fruit or Berry Compote

For this fruit topping, you can use strawberries, blackberries, blueberries, boysenberries, raspberries, peaches, nectarines, apricots, or a combination of fruits or berries. For the juice, you can use apple, cranberry, cran-apple, cran-raspberry, pomegranate, or a combination of juices. You might want to try several different ones or use whatever you have in the refrigerator or freezer. Here's one example just to show you the proportions.

Ingredients:
- 1 cup of cran-raspberry juice
- 1 Tbsp cornstarch
- 2 Tbsp honey
- 1 cup mixed berries (fresh or frozen)

Directions: Combine the juice and cornstarch in a small saucepan. Add the honey and cook over medium heat until the mixture boils and becomes clear. Add the berries and continue cooking for a minute or two, just until the berries are softened. Serve over pancakes, waffles, ice cream, cheese-cake or even cottage cheese or yogurt for a late night snack.

Liver Glycogen Yield per serving (2 Tbsp): ~ **5 - 6 grams**

Apple Cinnamon Compote with Brandy

This one is great for pancakes or waffles or as a sauce for a pork chop or pork loin roast. How's that for a versatile topping. It is included to give you one more variation for a fruit topping. (You will want to double this recipe if serving with sliced pork loin or pork chops. Folks will want more.)

Ingredients:
- 1 cup apple or orange juice
- 1 Tbsp cornstarch
- 2 Tbsp honey
- 1 cup sliced apples (cored and peeled) (Honey crisp apples are best when you can get them)
- 1 Tbsp butter

- 2-3 tsp cinnamon (how much depends on how much you like cinnamon)
- ¼ tsp nutmeg
- 1 Tbsp brandy (optional)

Directions: Place the honey, apples, butter, spices, and brandy and cook over medium heat for 15 to 20 minutes or until the apples are soft. Combine the juice and cornstarch and add to a saucepan and cook until thickened. Serve warm.

Liver Glycogen Yield per serving (¼ cup): ~ **7 - 8 grams**

Cheese

There are dozens of kinds and types of cheese that one can use for appetizers or snacks. We're talking about real cheese here, none of that imitation stuff. The reason that real cheese is emphasized should be obvious. Imitation or processed cheese contains more sugar (sucrose) than natural cheese and gets up to 50% of its total calories from carbohydrates. Real cheese contains from 5 to 15 times more protein per ounce than imitation cheese.

The liver glycogen yield from cheese comes mainly from the protein it contains. Some glycogen is also produced from lactose, a disaccharide made up of glucose and galactose, two sugars that form glycogen in the liver. We've included a few kinds of cheese here just to show you the liver glycogen yield from a single serving (~ 2 ounces).

Cheddar Cheese

Similar liver glycogen yield is obtained from most brick and hard cheeses including cheddar varieties, Colby, provolone, Parmesan, Monterey or jack, Gouda, Gruyere, mozzarella and Swiss cheeses. **Liver Glycogen Yield** per serving (2 oz): ~ **2 – 3 grams**

Couple any of the above cheeses with sliced apples, pears, or your favorite melon and you have a brain healthy snack or appetizer that delivers ~ **14 to 18 grams** of liver glycogen per serving.

Semi-soft Cheese

Feta cheese and other semi-soft cheeses like goat, bleu, Camembert, or Brie have just slightly less liver glycogen yield per serving than do the hard cheeses, primarily due to the lower amount of sugar and protein found in them. Of course you can always top a round of warm Brie with a honey and walnut glaze to add to the liver glycogen yield. **Liver Glycogen Yield** per serving (2 oz): ~ **3 grams**

Cream or Neufchatel Cheese

These soft cheeses produce less liver glycogen due to the smaller amount of protein per ounce that they contain. However, they make a great base for dips and spreads, especially when one adds honey. **Liver Glycogen Yield** per serving (2 oz): ~ **3 – 4 grams**

Crackers

Cheese and crackers – hard to beat as a mid-afternoon snack, but don't count on most baked cracker varieties to add much to the liver glycogen reserve. Crackers (and there are dozens of varieties) are made from various kinds of flour, all of which becomes glucose once digested. On reaching the blood stream, this glucose only contributes to the blood sugar total. The small amount of protein in a 1-2 ounce serving of crackers will net only 1 gram or so of liver glycogen, hardly enough to count.

For more recipes for appetizers using honey, go to www.foodnetwork.com or www.honey.com. Over 400 options can be found on these websites. The amount of Liver Glycogen Yield from each recipe will vary depending on the amount of honey used in each serving or portion.

Chapter 12 - Beverages

Iced Honey Coffee Energy Drink
  Ingredients:
- Coffee - 8 ounces freshly brewed strong roast regular or decaffeinated coffee (try different flavors to add variety)
- Milk - 2 - 4 ounces whole milk or 2%
- Honey - 2 ounces (2 Tbsp)
- Options: of course you can use any other flavors that you want but be cautious of the syrups and nondairy creamers. They may add flavor, but don't contribute much to liver glycogen yield. Instead, try a teaspoon of rum, vanilla or almond flavored extract for a real treat.

Directions: Dissolve honey in warm coffee. Pour into 32-ounce cup filled with ice. Add milk and stir. For a richer drink, use 2 ounces of half and half instead of milk.

Liver Glycogen Yield per serving (1 cups - 8 oz): ~ **15 grams** per cup.

[Note: this is a perfect energy drink to top off the liver glycogen reserve before and following exercise. In addition to the liver glycogen yield, the proteins from the milk will provide additional nutrition for muscles in the pre- and post-exercise period.]

Coffee or Tea with Honey
Honey may be used as a sweetener for both tea and coffee at any time of the day or evening. One ounce of cream would add less than a gram of liver glycogen yield when added to a cup of coffee or tea. **Liver Glycogen Yield** per serving (2 tsp honey in 8 oz of coffee or tea): **8 - 10 grams**
[**Note**: Heating honey to the temperature of drinkable tea or coffee does not alter the goodness of honey. The ratio of fructose to glucose is not changed. The natural enzymes in honey are all heat stable over brief periods of time. The small amount of advanced glycation end products (AGEs) like methylglyoxal (MGO) (which are potentially harmful to diabetics) formed when sugars are heated with proteins from pollen or milk products are not of significant dose to cause concern.]

Honey Watermelon Cooler
Ingredients:
- ¼ cup honey
- 3 cups watermelon juice
- 1 cup champagne or sparkling white wine (or substitute club soda)
- Ice

Directions: To make watermelon juice, place chunks of watermelon in blender, puree, and strain to get a clearer juice. Warm honey slightly with a bit of the watermelon juice so that it will dissolve easily. Add to watermelon juice. Pour juice over ice and add champagne or sparkling wine or club soda.

Liver Glycogen Yield per serving (6 ounces): **~ 12 grams**

The Beehive – a Honey of a Martini (not for Baptists) [66]
Ingredients:
- Ice cubes (about 1 cup)
- ½ cup pear vodka (4 ounces)
- Splash of cold water
- ¼ cup honey simple syrup (see directions below)
- ¼ cup lemon juice
- 2 to 3 pear slices for garnish

Directions: Place about one cup of ice in a cocktail shaker. Add vodka, a splash of water, simple syrup, and lemon juice. Cover and shake until well combined. Strain into chilled martini glasses. Garnish with pear slices and serve.

Liver Glycogen Yield per serving (4 ounces): **~ 8 grams**

To make honey simple syrup: gently heat 1 cup of honey and 1-cup water (total amounts may vary but be sure to use equal parts) in saucepan until honey is dissolved. Do not boil or use microwave. Cool completely before using. Honey simple syrup can be used in place of simple syrup made with sugar and water. Be sure to refrigerate leftover syrup.

RevHoney™ **Honey Drink**

This one requires no preparation or mixing. Just pop the top of the can and enjoy. *RevHoney*™ is available from stores across the Midwest or online at www.revhoney.com. There are a whopping 2 tablespoons of honey in every 16-oz can.

Liver Glycogen Yield per serving (8 ounces): ~ **15 grams**

Honey Lemonade or Limeade
Ingredients:
- ¾ cup Lemon or Lime juice
- 1 cup honey
- 1 cup water

Directions: To make the honey-lemon syrup, the proportions are simple. Just use equal amounts of honey and water (1 cup of each) and about ¾ cup of either fresh lemon or lime juice. Honey will dissolve in most acidic liquids like lemon or limejuice. But it does not dissolve well in water unless of course you heat the water. If you warm the mixture, use low heat and stir until the mixture is blended. Add ¼ cup of the honey-lemon syrup to 1 cup of water and pour over ice in a glass. Or add the whole batch of syrup to 2 ½ quarts of water, stir and pour over ice to serve.

Liver Glycogen Yield per serving (8 ounces): **1 - 2 grams**

More recipes for beverages using honey can be found in *The Buzz on Honey* by Marcella Richman (18) and at www.honey.com (44). The amount of Liver Glycogen Yield will vary depending on the ratio of ingredients. Remember, a tablespoon of honey will provide 15 – 17 grams of liver glycogen.

Chapter 13 - From Salads to Salsas

Salads

*T*ired of boring lettuce? Then read on for some liver-glycogen friendly, as well as tasty, alternatives. We'll give you the list of ingredients first, followed by a section on salad dressings, sauces and salsas and then offer a few specific menu suggestions.

Leafy greens. There are dozens of varieties to try: lettuce, bib lettuce, butter lettuce, arugula, spinach, romaine, dandelion and turnip greens to name a few. For ease of shopping and simplicity, try the seasonal salad mixes, pre-washed and mixed, available in bags or plastic boxes ready to use.

Salad Vegetables. Again the list is endless. Tomatoes (several varieties including heirloom tomatoes that can be sliced, diced, or wedged), celery (sliced thin or chopped) or celery root, jicama (crunchy and slightly sweet, cut in thin strips or shredded for slaw), cucumbers, carrots, bell peppers (red, orange, yellow, and green), onions (yellow, red, white, green), radishes, sprouts (bean, alfalfa, and others) and cabbage (red or white) and many varieties of hot peppers if you want to spice up your salads (Anaheim, jalapeño, poblano, Serrano, etc.).

Fruits. Melons (many varieties available year round plus seasonal favorites), apples, citrus (oranges, grapefruit in sections or wedges), pineapple, pears (at least seven or eight varieties), mango, papaya, bananas, blackberries, blueberries, raspberries, Marion berries, just to name a few.

Extras. Candied or dried fruit (cranberries, mango, papaya), nuts (sliced or slivered almonds), coconut, croutons (make them yourselves out of day old bread or leftover buns, sprinkle with olive oil, salt and pepper and toast in the oven) and many types of cheeses, shredded or sliced thin.

Salad Dressings

One of the best ways to avoid the unnecessary and excessive consumption of sucrose, HFCS, and preservatives is to avoid prepared salad dressings. It is so easy and healthful to make your own dressings with a few basic ingredients. Not only does it keep your refrigerator uncluttered by numerous bottles (I have counted as many as 13 different bottles of dressings by snooping in the refrigerators of unsuspecting friends and relatives, some of you may have more than 13 – you know who you are), but also tastes better, saves money, and provides a delightful relief from having to buy a favorite dressing or two or three for each member of the family (most of which stay on the refrigerator shelf for weeks or months).

Here are the basics, listed in no particular order. The Liver Glycogen Yield has been estimated for each based on the approximate amount that may be used in making a dressing.

- **Olive oil** or one of several preferred vegetable oils (canola, corn, safflower, etc.) or melted bacon fat
  Liver Glycogen Yield per serving (2 Tbsp): **0 grams** [Fats do not produce Liver Glycogen]
- **Yogurt** (Remember to buy only natural yogurt, not the non-fat or low-fat variety. Also skip the fruit flavored "light" or "low-fat" yogurts of which there are dozens of varieties. All of these contain sugar or HFCS or other sweeteners.)
  Liver Glycogen Yield per serving (1 cup): **~ 16 grams**
- **Mayonnaise** (real - not the imitation)
  Liver Glycogen Yield per serving (1 cup): **~ 8 grams**
- **Mustard** (stone ground or Dijon or another favorite variety)
  Liver Glycogen Yield per serving (1 Tbsp): **~ 1 gram**
- **Sour cream or buttermilk** (Don't forget the blue cheese or feta cheese crumbles.)
  Liver Glycogen Yield per serving (1 cup): **~ 11 gram**
- **Honey**. Honey is the only sweetener you will need to make any number of wonderful natural salad dressings for any type of salad. We'll give you some specific recipes later for those who are hesitant to experiment.
  Liver Glycogen Yield per serving (2 Tbsp): **~ 30 grams**

- **Some form of acid** such as a preferred distilled vinegar, apple cider vinegar, white or red wine vinegar or even balsamic vinegar, or citrus juices such as lemon, lime, orange or others. Unused pickle juice from the jar of sweet or dill pickles also makes a great addition to homemade salad dressings.
  Liver Glycogen Yield per serving (¼ cup): ~ **½ gram** for cider vinegar and ~ **4 grams** for orange juice

- **Spices and herbs.** Most of you will have a variety of spices in your spice cabinet already. Adding a few fresh herbs to your grocery list will not break the budget and will provide wonderful sensory and taste enhancements to your meals. Poppy seeds or other seeds are a good addition also. Basil, parsley (several varieties), cilantro, mint, dill, oregano, thyme, tarragon and chives are all available in small amounts. You can even buy organic if that is important to you, however, organically grown herbs are overrated and an unnecessary expense given the small amounts that one uses in dressings.
  Liver Glycogen Yield per serving 1 tsp – 1 Tbsp): No appreciable amount of liver glycogen is formed from these small amounts of herbs.

- Other aromatics such as garlic and onion, green onions and the zest from oranges, lemons or limes
  Liver Glycogen Yield per serving 1 tsp – 1 Tbsp): No appreciable amount of liver glycogen is formed from these amounts of aromatics.

- Salt and pepper

Some of you are already protesting, "That's not simple. I don't have the time to make a new dressing for every meal. And you have listed ten categories of items. Takes up over a page!"

So lets break it down into a few simple principles just to get started. You can make it more complicated as you discover a few things later.

Perhaps the simplest and most tasteful salad dressing for a basic lettuce salad can be made from two or three ingredients – yogurt and honey or sour cream and honey. Of course if you like mustard, you can add a little Dijon or stone-ground mustard (or both) to the yogurt and honey and have a wonderful honey-mustard dressing that is fresh and tangy and will be enjoyed by most. You can experiment with the proportions of each to get the desired sweetness or spiciness and even use mayonnaise and sour cream and/or yogurt. Each combination will give you a different bit of creaminess or flavor, but the dressing and the liver glycogen yield will be essentially the same.

Add tomatoes, and a bit of sliced red onion, sliced almonds, black olives, or chopped dried fruit bits to a lettuce mix and you have a wonderful compliment for any meal.

A simple yogurt and honey dressing for fruit salads is another two-ingredient dressing that is not only tasty but also healthy.

One thing to keep in mind when using honey in any dressing is that it is very hygroscopic. That means that it attracts or absorbs water. When sitting for even short periods of time uncovered, dressings made with honey will become more liquid or diluted, as the honey will absorb water from anything, including air. And when using a honey-based dressing on a fruit salad, the honey will pull water out of the fruit leaving you with more liquid at the bottom of the bowl. It is a good idea to add a honey-based dressing to a vegetable or fruit salad just before serving it or serve it on the side for addition just before eating.

When making an oil-based dressing, here are some suggestions to keep in mind. Start with an acid (choice of vinegar or citrus juice or combination) and add honey (honey will dissolve well in vinegar or acidic juices), sweeten to taste, then add your choice of oil in a one-to-one or up to a one-to-two ratio, whisking the oil into the vinegar and honey mixture.

You may also add mustard or mayo to this to achieve the desired amount of creaminess, taste or texture. Then add salt and pepper to taste and finely chopped herbs that complement the other ingredients in the salad. This works great for pasta salads. Just add some chopped red and yellow peppers, a few black olives, pimentos, diced roasted red peppers, or a sliced red onion and a few chives or chopped green onions and you have a great pasta salad. Add some sliced cured meats like pepperoni, ham, prosciutto, or fried pancetta and you have a meal in itself. For a variation, add chopped tomatoes, goat cheese or blue cheese crumbles and some large homemade croutons made from left over day-old bread sprinkled with olive oil, salt and pepper and toasted in the oven.

Another suggestion is to keep brief notes on pro-portions and combinations. List the likes and dislikes of your family for the next time around. Disregard the unfavorable attempts and keep the ones they rave about (and they will)!

Simple Salad Dressing Recipes

Basic Vinaigrette

Generally, the ratio of acid (choice of vinegar or citrus juice or combination of both) to oil will be about 1:1 or 1:2 or more. So make it how you like it and don't be a slave to a formula. Add chopped green onions, chopped fresh herbs, salt and pepper to taste and whisk.

Here is a simple variation made with honey.

Honey Vinaigrette
Ingredients:
- 2 Tbsp vinegar
- 1 teaspoon Dijon mustard or stone ground mustard (or both)
- Shallot (or green onion) minced or chopped fine
- ¼ teaspoon salt
- Fresh ground pepper
- 1 Tbsp honey
- 4-6 Tbsp olive oil

Directions: Place first five ingredients in bowl. Whisk in 4-6 Tbsp of olive oil until mixture is smooth and creamy.

Liver Glycogen Yield per serving (2 Tbsp): **3 - 4 grams**

Basic Honey Mustard Dressing
Ingredients:
- 1 cup of yogurt, sour cream, or mayonnaise (or a combination of any two totaling a cup)
- 2 Tablespoons of honey

- Add 1 Tablespoon of Dijon or stone ground mustard (or a combination of both). Even plain yellow mustard works great
- Variations: 1 tsp of parsley, cilantro, dill, mint, or tarragon - finely chopped; 2 Tbsp parmesan cheese

Directions: Combine and mix well.
Liver Glycogen Yield per serving (2 Tbsp): **3 – 4 grams**

Honey French Dressing[67]
Ingredients:
- ¾ cup salad oil
- ¼ cup vinegar or lemon juice
- ½ tsp paprika
- ½ tsp salt
- 2 tsp yellow mustard (or ½ tsp dry mustard)
- Dash cayenne pepper
- ¼ cup honey

Directions: Place all ingredients in a blender and pulse until combined.
Liver Glycogen Yield per serving (2 Tbsp): ~ **6 – 7 grams**

Honey Russian Dressing[68]
Ingredients:
- ½ cup honey
- 1 cup salad oil
- ½ tsp salt
- 1/3 cup chili sauce (or use 1/3 cup home-made catsup and 2 tsp chili powder)
- ½ cup vinegar
- 1 medium onion grated
- 1 Tbsp Worcestershire

Directions: Place all ingredients in a blender and pulse until blended

Liver Glycogen Yield per serving (2 Tbsp): ~ 8 grams

Basic Creamy Dressing for Fruit Salads
Ingredients:
- 1 cup of yogurt or sour cream
- 2 Tablespoons of honey
- Variations:
- 1 tsp of mint leaves - finely chopped
- 1 tsp of orange or lime zest

Directions: Combine and add to fruit just before serving.

Note: If you are using yogurt, be sure to use regular yogurt or Greek yogurt for this, not low fat yogurt! You can even place regular yogurt in a strainer lined with a paper towel for 30 minutes to let more of the liquid drain out to give you a thicker dressing.

Liver Glycogen Yield per serving (2 Tbsp): **5 - 6 grams**

Panzanella - Italian Bread Salad
A great way to use up bread from the honey sourdough loaf. Or you can use crusty French bread. This recipe is a good illustration of how to boost the liver glycogen yield using something as simple as bread and vegetables. It's a meal in itself! Makes about 4 servings.

Ingredients:
- 3 cups of bread cubes (1" pieces of sourdough or French bread)
- Olive oil for toasting the bread cubes
- Salt and pepper
- ½ red bell pepper, ½ yellow bell pepper diced in ½" pieces

- 1 cup cucumber, peeled, seeded and diced (may use English cucumber without peeling or seeding if you want)
- ½ cup red onion, thinly sliced
- 1 cup tomatoes, use cherry, grape or Roma tomatoes cut in half or smaller pieces
- 1 cup fresh Mozzarella cheese, cut into ½ inch cubes (use Feta cheese or even blue cheese crumbles if you prefer)
- 2 cloves garlic minced or finely diced
- 1 avocado, pitted and diced
- 3 Tbsp fresh basil leaves, julienned or chopped
- 1 Tbsp Italian parsley, finely chopped
- 1 Tbsp capers (optional)
- ¼ cup red wine vinegar
- ¼ cup honey
- ¼ cup olive oil

Directions: Cube the bread and place on a cookie sheet. Drizzle with olive oil, salt and pepper and toast in the oven at 450⁰ F until golden brown, or you may toast the cubes in a hot skillet until crusty and brown. Set aside and let cool. Combine the vegetables, cheese, basil and parsley and toss lightly. To make the dressing, whisk the vinegar, honey and olive oil in a small bowl until well combined. When ready to serve, toss the browned croutons with the vegetables and herbs and the dressing. Season to taste with salt and fresh cracked pepper.

Liver Glycogen Yield per serving (1 ½ - 2 cups): ~ **17 - 23 grams**

Mediterranean Salad Variation

This is similar to Panzanella or Italian bread salad above, but contains meats and pasta and more veggies.

Ingredients:

- ½ cup each of Prosciutto, salami, pepperoni or smoked ham, sliced or diced (Use about 1 ½ cups total)
- 2 cups of cooked orzo, chick peas, drained or cooked spiral pasta, drained
- 1 cup roasted red bell peppers, diced and/or ½ red bell pepper, ½ yellow bell pepper diced in ½" pieces
- 1 cup cucumber, peeled, seeded and diced (may use English cucumber without peeling or seeding if you want)
- ½ cup red onion, thinly sliced
- 1 cup tomatoes, use cherry, grape or Roma tomatoes cut in half or smaller pieces
- 1 cup fresh Mozzarella cheese, cut into ½ inch cubes (use Feta cheese or even blue cheese crumbles if you prefer)
- 1 avocado, pitted and diced
- 2 cloves garlic minced, finely diced or grated
- ¼ cup red wine vinegar
- ¼ cup honey
- ¼ cup olive oil
- Salt and pepper
- 3 Tbsp fresh basil leaves, julienned or chopped
- 1 Tbsp Italian parsley, finely chopped
- 1 Tbsp capers (optional)

Directions: Combine the diced meats, vegetables, cheese, orzo (chick peas or pasta) and herbs. Toss lightly with the dressing when ready to serve.

To make the Dressing: Combine the vinegar, honey and olive oil and whisk until smooth. Season with salt, fresh cracked pepper and basil or Italian parsley.

Liver Glycogen Yield per serving (1 ½ - 2 cups): ~ **25 – 30 grams**

Sauces and Salsas

Tomato Sauce.

Making your own basic sauces from fresh ingredients is another place where one can avoid excess sugar and HFCS and improve the taste. This basic tomato sauce can be used for anything from spaghetti to pizza sauce to fresh tomato bisque with a few variations.

Ingredients:
- 2 cups whole fresh tomatoes (Use any type that are seasonal or inexpensive such as Roma, cherry, vine-ripened; large, medium or small; or even canned tomatoes)
- 1 medium onion, yellow or white, Maui or Vandalia, diced
- 2 garlic cloves, minced or chopped fine if you have them, or use 1 teaspoon garlic powder
- 1 cup yellow or red bell pepper, seeded and chopped
- Salt and pepper to taste
- 2 - 4 Tbsp honey
- 1 Tbsp olive oil / butter

Directions:

Sauté the onion in 1 Tbsp olive oil or butter in a saucepan over medium heat for 5 minutes. Add garlic and season with salt and pepper. Add tomatoes and bell peppers. For added flavor, roast fresh whole tomatoes and bell peppers in the oven at 375⁰ F for 30 minutes before adding to sauce pan. Add 2 - 4 Tbsp honey. When mixture is hot and bubbly, puree with an emersion blender (off of the stove) or place warm mixture into a blender or food processor and puree until smooth.

Store in an airtight container or jar in the refrigerator until use. Keeps 3 - 4 weeks or longer.
Liver Glycogen Yield per serving (½ cup): **~ 7 grams** [Note: the use of honey here is not intended to make a sweet sauce but rather to use just enough to balance the acidity of the tomatoes.]

Tomato Bisque

For a basic **tomato bisque,** use a little basal and oregano or add 1 tsp of anchovy paste. Warm 4 cups of the basic tomato sauce over medium heat until boiling. Reduce heat and add 1 cup of cream or half and half. Stir and warm just to near boiling again. Add a dollop of sour cream and sprinkle with chopped green onions or chives or finely chopped fresh mint leaves and serve. Makes 4 servings.
Liver Glycogen Yield per serving (1 ½ cup): **15 - 20 grams**

Pizza Sauce

For a basic **pizza sauce,** add 2 Tbsp of tomato paste to 1 cup of basic tomato sauce. Season with a 1 tsp of dried basal, 1 tsp of dried oregano, 1 tsp of salt and 1 tsp fresh ground pepper.
Liver Glycogen Yield per serving (½ cup): **~ 5 grams**

Spaghetti Sauce

For **spaghetti sauce,** add 4 Tbsp of tomato paste to 4 cups of basic tomato sauce. Season with a 1 – 2 tsp of dried basal, 1 Tsp of dried oregano, 1 tsp of salt and 1 tsp fresh ground pepper or use 1 ½ - 2 Tbsp of Italian seasoning. [Note: Homemade spaghetti sauce gets better the longer it simmers, even up to 1 or 2 hours] Add pre-cooked meatballs or sautéed Italian sausage and simmer until meatballs and sauce are warm throughout. Serve over spaghetti or linguini noodles or other preferred pasta. **Liver Glycogen Yield** per serving (1 cups): **~ 10 grams**

Homemade Catsup

This recipe will surprise you with its liver glycogen yield per serving and wonderful taste. No longer will you think of catsup as just having a lot of sugar! This one is healthy and full of fructose and glucose in proper proportions.

Ingredients:

- 3 or 4 vine ripened tomatoes, quartered and seeded (should have about 24 ounces or about 3 cups) OR
- 3 cups of canned whole tomatoes OR a combination of both totaling 3 cups
- ½ onion (about 1/2 cup), diced
- ¾ cup tomato paste (6 ounces)
- ¾ cup honey (6 ounces)
- ½ cup vinegar (4 ounces)
- 1 Tbsp Worcestershire sauce
- 1 Tbsp corn starch in 1 Tbsp of cold water (optional, depending on the water content of tomatoes)
- 2 tsp salt
- 1 tsp onion powder
- 1 tsp garlic powder

Directions: Process tomatoes and onions in a food processor until smooth and blended (1 to 2 minutes). (Or if you prefer, place all ingredients in a saucepan, heat to boiling. Remove from heat and puree using an emersion blender. Return to heat and cook on medium heat the 20 - 30 minutes.) Place mixture in a saucepan and add tomato paste, honey, vinegar, Worcestershire sauce and spices. Bring to boil over medium heat, then reduce heat and simmer, stirring frequently, for about 20 - 30 minutes until catsup is reduced and thickened. Add the cornstarch slurry at the last minute or so of cooking. (The cornstarch will keep the catsup from separating as it sits.) Cool and pour into sealable container (preferably glass) and keep in refrigerator. Shake well before serving. **Liver Glycogen Yield** per serving (2 Tbsp): ~ **8 grams**

Honey BBQ Sauce

There are dozens of combinations of ingredients that can go into a great BBQ sauce. Don't be afraid to experiment with these basic ingredients to come up with one that suits your tastes. Or you can start with a store bought sauce and spice it up. This recipe makes about 3 cups but you can easily double it and keep it in the refrigerator to use later.

Ingredients:
- 2 cups homemade catsup
- ¼ cup vinegar
- ¼ cup honey
- ¼ cup dark molasses (or use ¼ cup dark brown sugar)
- 1 Tbsp onion powder (or use ¼ cup finely chopped or minced onion)
- 1 Tbsp garlic powder (or use 2 or 3 cloves fresh garlic, finely chopped or minced)

- 1 tsp cumin
- 1 Tbsp chili powder (more or less to taste)
- 1 Tbsp Worcestershire sauce

Directions: Place all ingredients in a saucepan and heat over medium heat for 15 - 20 minutes. Cool and place in glass container with a sealable lid. Store in refrigerator.

Liver Glycogen Yield per serving (2 Tbsp): **~ 10 grams**

Enchilada Sauce
Ingredients:
- 1 cup basic tomato sauce
- ½ can (2 Tbsp) of green chilies
- 1 Tbsp of pickled jalapeno pepper slices if desired

Directions: Heat all ingredients together in a small pan. Blend with an emersion blender or place in a blender and mix until smooth.

Liver Glycogen Yield per serving (2 Tbsp): **~ 2 grams**

Mango Salsa
This makes a great salsa for chicken, fish, or to use as a dip for chips as an appetizer.

Ingredients:
- 2 - 3 whole ripe mangos
- ½ cup red onion, finely diced
- 2 Tbsp chopped green onion
- 2 Tbsp green pepper diced
- 2 Tbsp red pepper diced
- 1 Tbsp red wine vinegar (or use any kind you prefer)
- 2 - 3 Tbsp honey
- 1 Tbsp grated ginger root
- 1 Tbsp fresh basil, chopped fine

- 1 Tbsp chopped mint leaves (optional)
- Salt and pepper if desired

Directions: Slice the mangos vertically along either side of the center pit or use one of those cool mango slicers if you have one. With the skin or peel on still on, cut diagonal marks into the flesh side of each mango half with a paring knife being careful not to cut through the skin (or your hand). Repeat cutting at 90^0 to form diamond shaped sections. Remove mango sections with a spoon and place in small bowl. Add other ingredients and stir lightly.

As we have said before, the honey will "dehydrate" the fruit and cause the salsa to have more liquid the longer it sits. So this salsa is best made the day that you want to use it.

Liver Glycogen Yield per serving (2 Tbsp): **9 – 10 grams**

Pickled Cauliflower and Pepper Relish
Ingredients:
- 1 jar of pickled cauliflower and peppers, drained
- ½ cup of green olives with pimentos
- 2 Tbsp honey

Directions: Place the jar of pickled vegetables and olives in a food processor with the honey. Pulse a few times to finely chop the vegetables. No need to puree.

Liver Glycogen Yield per serving (2 Tbsp): **2 – 3 grams**

[Note: this is an easy way to make a quick relish for sandwiches. There are several varieties of pickled vegetables. Choose your favorite.]

The Buzz on Honey has a great section on "Salads and Sides" that includes recipes for many different kinds of salads using honey. Here are a few just to give you ideas:

- Apple Yogurt Salad
- Chicken Waldorf Salad
- Coleslaw with horseradish, nuts and honey
- Honey Almond Brie
- Honey Carrot Ambrosia
- Fruit and Wild Rice Salad
- Hawaiian Chicken Salad
- Oriental Noodle Salad
- Strawberry-Orange-Spinach Salad

In addition, Marcella includes the recipes for over a dozen dressings, spreads and dips made with honey, everything from Honey Kiwi Spread to Parisian Fruit Dressing to Raspberry Vinaigrette.

Chapter 14 - Breads

Wheat Honey Sourdough

I know! It's not logical to add honey to sourdough bread! Just try it. You will love it. From this basic recipe you can make a beautiful rounded loaf, a long crusty loaf, a traditional loaf using a bread pan, or dinner rolls in several shapes.

Ingredients:

- 1 ¼ cup sourdough starter (at room temperature) (recipe follows)
- ½ to ¾ cup water (use warm water if your sour dough starter is cold or you do not have enough time or patience to let it come to room temperature). Amount of water will vary depending on weather and altitude. Use just enough to make a soft pliable dough. Start with ½ cup and add more as needed.
- 1 ½ cup whole wheat flour
- 1 ½ cup bread flour (or for a lighter bread use 1 cup of whole wheat flour to 2 cups of bread flour)
- ¼ cup honey
- 1 tsp salt

- 1 ¼ - 1 ½ tsp bread machine (fast acting or rapid rising) yeast (if you are cooking at altitude above 6000 ft as in Colorado or on Mt Rainier in Washington, reduce the amount of yeast by ¼ to ½ tsp.)
- Options: add ¼ cup of sunflower seeds and or ¼ cup of wheat germ

Directions: Add all ingredients together, combine in bread machine on "dough" cycle and mix for 20 minutes or knead for 10 to 15 minutes on a floured counter or until dough is smooth and of even consistency. Cover and let rise for 1 to 1 ½ hours in a warm spot or if using a bread machine, let dough rise in the bread machine for an hour or through the dough cycle.

Single loaf. Place dough on a floured sheet pan that you have first sprayed lightly with a non-stick spray and shape into round loaf or long loaf, or place in a greased and floured bread pan. Cover and let rise for an hour. Brush with melted butter or olive oil for a crispier crust and bake in a 400⁰ F (425⁰ F at altitudes above 6000 feet) oven for 22-25 minutes or until golden brown.
Liver Glycogen Yield per serving (1 slice = 30 grams): ~ **2 grams**

Dinner rolls. After dough has risen for the first hour or so, pinch off small amounts of dough and roll into one-inch balls. Place three dough balls in each section of a muffin tin. Let rise for another hour or until the dough fills the muffin tin sections. Bake at 400° F for 18 to 20 minutes or until brown.
Liver Glycogen Yield per serving (1 roll = 30 grams): ~ **2 grams**

Sour Dough Starter
  Ingredients:
- 1 tsp fast acting or bread machine yeast
- ¼ cup warm water (~ 110⁰ F or warm tap water)
- ¾ cup milk
- 1 cup bread flour

Directions: Dissolve the yeast in the warm water in a quart glass jar and add the milk. Gradually stir in the flour and mix well until smooth. Cover with a towel and let stand in a warm, draft-free place (80⁰ to 85⁰ F). Bubbles will begin to appear in about 24 hours as the starter begins to ferment.

When fermentation has begun, stir well, then cover with a lid and let stand an additional 2-3 days or until the starter is quite foamy (bubbly). Stir again and cover with lid and screw top ring. Keep in refrigerator until ready to use.

To replenish starter after each use, add ¾ to 1 cup of milk and ¾ to 1-cup bread flour. Mix thoroughly and let stand on counter top for an hour or so. Then replace the lid firmly and refrigerate until next use. Starter will expand some even while in the refrigerator.

Banana Nut-N-Honey Bread
  Ingredients:
- 1 ½ cup whole wheat flour
- ½ cup bread flour
- 1 teaspoon baking soda
- ½ teaspoon salt
- 2 eggs
- 1 teaspoon vanilla extract
- ½ cup (1 stick) butter
- 1 cup honey
- 3 ripe bananas (mashed) (about 1 cup)

- 1 cup pecans or walnuts

Directions: Preheat oven to 350⁰ F. Grease baking pan with butter.

Combine whole-wheat flour, bread flour, baking soda and salt together in a bowl. In a small bowl, beat the eggs and vanilla together. In a mixing bowl, cream the butter and honey together until light and fluffy. Slowly add the egg mixture to the creamed butter and mix until well incorporated. Add the mashed bananas and mix well. (The mixture will appear to be lumpy or curdled.) Remove mixing bowl from mixer and fold in the flour a bit at a time. Fold in the nuts. The batter will be thick. No need to over mix. Pour batter into the prepared baking pan and bake for 55 to 60 minutes or until a cake tester (toothpick) inserted into the center of the loaf comes out clean. Let the loaf cool for 10 minutes on a wire rack before turning out. When cool, wrap the loaf with plastic wrap.

A little softened cream cheese mixed with honey (or honey butter, recipe follows) makes a wonderful spread for this banana bread!

Liver Glycogen Yield per serving (1 slice): **18 – 20 grams**

Honey Butter

This is a basic staple for a well-set table. Use it on pancakes, toast, muffins, cornbread, even over steamed vegetables. Try one of the variations to serve over salmon or other fish.

Ingredients:
- 2 sticks butter (1 cup) at room temperature
- ½ cup honey
- 1 tsp orange (or lemon) zest

Directions: Whip the butter until fluffy and light. Add the honey and the zest and continue whipping until well combined. Place in a ramekin and cover with plastic wrap. Chill until firm. Before serving, bring to room temperature or until butter softens a bit.

Variations: add a teaspoon of finely chopped garlic, shallots or add ½ tsp of dried oregano or dried basil or mint.

Liver Glycogen Yield per serving (1 Tbsp): **~4-5 grams**

Peanut Butter Honey Bread[69]
Ingredients:
- 2 cups all-purpose flour
- 4 teaspoons baking powder
- 1 tsp salt
- ½ cup peanut butter
- 1/3 cup honey
- 1 ½ cup milk

Directions: Sift together flour, baking powder and salt. Blend peanut butter and honey and add to the flour mixture along with the milk, gradually forming soft dough. Pour into a greased pan and bake at 350⁰ F for 1 hour.

Liver Glycogen Yield per serving (1 slice): **~7-8 grams**

Honey Orange Muffins
Ingredients:
- ½ cup all-purpose flour
- ½ tsp salt
- 2 tsp baking powder
- ½ cup whole wheat flour
- 1 egg, beaten
- ¼ cup orange juice
- 1 tsp orange zest
- ½ cup honey
- 3 Tbsp melted butter or shortening

Directions: Sift together first 3 ingredients. Add whole-wheat flour and mix thoroughly. Combine egg, orange juice, orange zest, honey and butter or shortening. Add wet ingredients to dry ingredients, stirring only enough to dampen all the flour. Pour or spoon into muffin pans being careful not to fill more than 2/3 of the way. Bake at 400⁰ F for 15 to 20 minutes or until browned. Cool muffins slightly for 5 minutes before turning out.

Liver Glycogen Yield per serving (1 muffin): ~ **10 - 12 grams**

Cornbread and variations

This cornbread goes great with soups and chili. You can make it with shredded cheese, green chilies, or both. Cornbread is a great "carrier" for extra honey!

Ingredients:
- 1 cup cornmeal
- 1 cup bread flour
- 1 tsp baking powder
- 1 tsp baking soda
- ½ cup honey
- ½ cup vegetable oil (also good with ¼ cup bacon fat and ¼ vegetable oil)
- 2 large eggs, whisked slightly
- 1 ¼ cup buttermilk
- Optional: 7 oz can of diced green chilies, ½ cup of grated cheese

Directions: Mix the dry ingredients together in a large mixing bowl. In another bowl combine the honey, vegetable oil, eggs and buttermilk. Add the wet ingredients to the dry cornmeal mixture and stir gently until the batter is smooth and moistened. No need to over mix.

Pour batter into a buttered 8 inch round non-stick baking pan (square is OK too, don't stress over this one). Place in a preheated oven at 375⁰ F for 25 minutes or until lightly browned. Serve warm with butter and honey.

Liver Glycogen Yield per serving (2x3" piece or ~ 60 grams): ~ **5 - 6 grams**

[Note: the liver glycogen yield is mostly from the honey and buttermilk. The other carbohydrates from the corn meal and flour are converted to glucose after ingestion.]

Other Breads and Baked Goods

The Liver Glycogen Yield from the breads and baked goods listed below will vary from ~ 8 - 20 grams per slice depending on the amount of honey in each recipe. A half-cup of honey adds about 120 grams of LGY to each recipe. If each recipe makes a loaf consisting of 16 slices, each slice will contribute about 8 grams of liver glycogen plus the liver glycogen available from other fruit, vegetables and nuts.

The recipes for these delicious baked goods can be found at the National Honey Board's official website (www.honey.com).

- Apricot Honey Bread
- Cinnamon Honey Glazed Sticky Buns
- Cranberry Muffins
- Currant Scone
- Guava Cheesecake
- Holiday Scone Mix
- Honey Mango Margarita Cupcakes
- Honey Pecan Bran Muffins
- Orange Honey Almond Muffins

- Poppy Seed Roll
- Pumpkin Muffins with Cream Cheese Frosting

Many more recipes using honey are included in Marcella Richman's cookbook, *The Buzz on Honey*. I have included the titles here just to give you ideas.

- Apple Graham Muffins
- Apricot and Honey Rye Bread
- Honey Bran Muffins
- Blueberry Muffins
- Honey Buns
- Honey Date Bread
- Honey Orange Rolls
- Honey Zucchini Bread
- Pineapple-Orange-Banana Bread
- Pumpkin Bread

Included with the recipes in Marcella's cookbook are these wonderful ideas for spreads, sauces, and jams using honey:

- Almond Sauce
- Honey Apple Butter
- Apricot Honey Freezer Jam
- Apricot Pineapple Butter
- Berry Butter
- Cream Cheese Honey Almond Spread
- Several Varieties of Honey Butter
- Honey Peach Jam
- Honey Strawberry Jam
- Plum Butter
- Swiss Honey Butter
- Whipped Honey Butter

Chapter 15 - Meats

Chicken

Honey Orange Glaze for Chicken
  Ingredients:
- 1 Tbsp olive oil
- 1 Tbsp shallots, finely chopped (or use onions)
- ½ cup honey
- ¼ cup Balsamic vinegar
- 1 cup orange juice
- 1 Tbsp orange zest (zest from 1 orange)
- 1 Tbsp grated ginger
- ½ cup orange marmalade

Directions: To make the glaze, sauté the shallots (or onions) until soft in a small saucepan in the olive oil. Add other ingredients for glaze and bring to a boil. Lower heat to medium. Reduce glaze by about 50% (or about 15 minutes). Brush on chicken before grilling or baking in the oven after the chicken is partially cooked. If using a rotisserie, place whole chicken on the spit and drizzle with olive oil, salt and pepper. Cook chicken over even heat while rotating until internal temperature reaches 140^0 F (about 1 hour to 1 ½ hours). During last 30 to 45 minutes of cooking, brush chicken with glaze every 10 to 15 minutes. If roasting whole chicken in the oven, drizzle with olive oil and season well with salt and pepper. Roast for 1 hour before basting with glaze. Baste every 15 minutes or until internal temperature of chicken reaches 160 - 165^0 F.

This glaze can be used for chicken pieces, breasts or thighs, whole chicken for rotisserie or roasting, split and flattened chicken for grilling or oven roasting.

For a split and flattened chicken, use sharp kitchen shears to remove the backbone of one whole chicken by cutting along each side of the spine. Flatten chicken by pulling the sides apart. Place the whole chicken, skin side up on cutting board or counter and pushing down gently until the breast and ribs loosen and flatten out. Season with olive oil and salt and pepper. Brown chicken on both sides in a large heavy skillet (cast iron is best). Brush chicken with glaze and finish cooking chicken (in the skillet) in the oven at 350^0 F for 30 minutes.

Liver Glycogen Yield per serving of glazed chicken: **15 - 40 grams**.

[Note: Approximately 75 - 80 % of the amino acids in chicken (both dark and breast meat) can be used by the liver to make liver glycogen, but when a mixed carbohydrate meal is consumed with protein, most of the immediate liver glycogen made will come from fructose and glucose in the carbohydrates. One-half of a roasted chicken will provide about 35 to 40 grams of amino acids that may be used to form liver glycogen. A smaller 6-ounce serving of chicken will provide about 15 grams of amino acids that may be used to form liver glycogen. Again, the actual amount of liver glycogen formed from the amino acids will depend more on the amount of fructose and glucose from carbohydrates consumed with the chicken.]

Honey Lime Chicken Enchiladas (recipe submitted by Carolyn Hock)
   Ingredients:
- 6 Tbsp honey
- 5 Tbsp limejuice (juice from 1 large lime)
- 1 Tbsp chili powder
- ½ tsp garlic powder
- 3 cups chicken, cooked and shredded (or 2 – 3 chicken breasts)
- 8 flour tortillas
- 16 oz Monterey jack cheese, shredded
- 16 oz green enchilada sauce
- 1 cup heavy cream or sour cream

Directions: Mix the honey, limejuice, chili powder and garlic powder and toss with the shredded chicken. Let it marinate for at least ½ hour at room temperature (or keep in the refrigerator several hours). Pour about ½ cup of the enchilada sauce on the bottom of a 9 X 13" baking pan. Fill the flour tortillas with the chicken and shredded cheese, roll up and place in the baking dish. Reserve about 1 cup of the cheese to sprinkle on top of the enchiladas. Mix the remaining enchilada sauce with the cream and any leftover marinade. Pour the sauce on top of the enchiladas and sprinkle with the grated cheese. Bake at 350⁰ F for 30 minutes or until brown on top. **Liver Glycogen Yield** per serving (1 enchilada): **32 – 35 grams**

Crockpot Honey Sesame Chicken (recipe submitted by Carolyn Hock)
  Ingredients:
  - 5 – 6 boneless chicken thighs or 2 - 3 chicken breasts
  - 1 cup honey
  - Salt and pepper
  - ½ cup low sodium soy sauce
  - ¼ cup homemade catsup
  - 2 Tbsp vegetable oil
  - ½ cup diced onion
  - 2 cloves garlic, minced
  - ¼ tsp red pepper flakes
  - Cornstarch
  - Sesame seeds

Directions: Place the chicken in the crock-pot and season with salt and pepper. Combine the honey, soy sauce, catsup, oil, onion, garlic, and red pepper flakes in a small bowl, stir well and pour over the chicken. Cook on low for 3 - 4 hours or on high for 1 ½ to 2 hours. Remove the chicken from the crock-pot and cut into chunks. Combine the cornstarch with cold water and whisk it into the sauce in the crockpot. Return the cut up chicken to the crockpot, sprinkle with 1 Tbsp of sesame seeds, stir gently and keep on low or warm until ready to serve. Serve over cooked white rice and sprinkle with additional sesame seeds.

Liver Glycogen Yield per serving (about 1 ½ cups with rice): **75 - 80 grams**

Other Honey and Chicken Recipe Options (from honey.com)
  - Almond Chicken with Honey Lime Sauce
  - Apricot Glazed Chicken

- Spicy Honey Grilled Chicken
- Caribbean Chicken with Honey Pineapple Sauce
- Honey-Spiced Chicken with Mango
- Far East Chicken Strips with Fruit
- Chicken Fingers with Honey Mustard Dipping Sauce
- Grilled Honey Bourbon Chicken
- Honey Ginger Roasted Chicken
- One Skillet Chicken and Vegetables
- Thai Honey Chicken Wings
- Teriyaki Chicken with Honey and Sesame Seeds

Liver Glycogen Yield per serving: Each cup of chicken will provide about **20 to 25 grams** of liver glycogen. Each Tbsp of honey will add another **15 to 17 grams**. A good estimate of LGY per serving from each of these recipes would be **35 to 40 grams**, about ½ of the total storage capacity of the liver.

Duck Recipes (from honey.com)
- Duck Breasts with Raspberry Honey Glaze
- Duck Breast with Tangy Honey Sauce

Liver Glycogen Yield per serving (½ duck breast): ~ **35 – 40 grams**

Pork

Crockpot Honey Roast Pork (recipe submitted by Carolyn Hock)
Ingredients:
- 3 pound boneless pork roast (or pork butt)
- 1 cup grated Parmesan Cheese
- ½ cup honey
- 3 Tbsp soy sauce

- 2 Tbsp dried basil
- 2 Tbsp minced garlic
- 2 Tbsp olive oil
- ½ tsp salt
- 2 Tbsp cornstarch
- ¼ cup cold water

Directions: Spray crockpot or slow cooker with non-stick cooking spray. Place pork roast in crockpot.

In a small bowl, combine the cheese, honey, soy sauce, basil, garlic, oil, and salt. Pour over roast. Cover and cook for 6 – 7 hours or until inserted meat thermometer reads 160^0 F.

Remove meat to a serving platter and keep warm.

Skim fat from cooking juices and transfer to a small saucepan. Bring liquid to a boil.

Combine cornstarch and water and add to the liquid in the saucepan and stir. Bring to a boil, reduce heat and stir until sauce has thickened. Serve with portions of the roast.

Liver Glycogen Yield per serving (about 100 grams or a little over 3 oz. with sauce): **28 – 30 grams**

More Pork and Ham Recipes (from honey.com)
- Baked Honey Ham
- Grilled Pork Tenderloins with Rich Honey Port Sauce
- Honey Glazed Pork Tenderloin with Onions
- Honey Mustard Glazed Pork Chop
- Margarita Ribs
- Pulled Pork Shoulder with Honey BBQ sauce
- Stuffed Pork Roast with Apples and Cinnamon
- Sweet and Spicy Pork Ribs
- Honey Apple Chutney Pork Chops

Liver Glycogen Yield per serving (100 grams or a little over 3 oz.): ~ **30 – 32 grams**

Seafood

Tilapia Filets with Mango Salsa
Ingredients:
- 4 – 6 frozen or fresh tilapia filets
- Olive oil
- Salt and pepper
- Mango Salsa (see recipe on page 188)

Directions: Drizzle a small amount of olive oil over filets, season with salt and pepper, and fry in olive oil until golden brown (do not over cook). Serve with Mango salsa.

Liver Glycogen Yield per serving (100 grams or a little over 3 oz. of fish with 2 Tbsp mango salsa): ~ **24 grams**

More Seafood Recipes (from honey.com)
- Asian Honey Grilled Prawns
- Salmon with Honey Glaze
- Cod or Catfish Filets with Honey Dipping Sauce
- Scallops with Honey-lime Marinade
- Honey Glazed Shrimp
- Sweet Spicy Salmon with Honey Mango Salsa

Liver Glycogen Yield per serving (100 grams or a little over 3 oz.): ranges from ~ **15 – 18 grams** for shrimp and prawns to ~ **35 grams** for salmon with honey mango salsa

Beef

Meatloaf with Honey and Pine Nuts (adapted from honey.com)
Ingredients:
- 5 Tbsp honey

- 2 lbs ground chuck or 1 lb each of ground veal and ground pork
- 1 cup chopped onion
- ½ cup breadcrumbs softened in ½ cup milk
- 2 eggs
- 1/3 cup pine nuts
- ½ cup sun-dried tomatoes, chopped
- 1 Tbsp thyme
- 1 ½ tsp cumin
- 1 ½ tsp black pepper

Directions: Combine 4 Tbsp (¼ cup) of honey with al other ingredients and mix evenly. Place mixture into a 9 x 5-inch pan. Drizzle remaining Tbsp of honey over the meatloaf and spread to cover top. Bake uncovered at 400⁰ F for 50 to 60 minutes. Let rest 5 minutes before slicing.

Liver Glycogen Yield per serving (3 oz): **20 grams**

More Beef Recipes (from honey.com)
- Burgers with Honey Pineapple Chutney
- Honey-bronzed Brisket
- Chinese Beef and Tomatoes
- Meatloaf with Honey and Pine Nuts
- Korean Style Beef (Flank Steak)
- Sirloin Steaks with Texas-Style Honey BBQ Rub

Liver Glycogen Yield per serving (100 grams or a little over 3 oz.): **19 – 22 grams** from beef alone. Another **15 – 18 grams** of liver glycogen will be formed from the honey and other ingredients listed for a total of **34 – 40 grams** per serving.

Spaghetti and Meatballs

This classic favorite provides a huge amount of liver glycogen per serving because of the fructose-glucose rich sauce and the amino acids from the

meatballs. Honey is added not to make a sweet sauce but to balance the acidy of the tomatoes.
Ingredients:
- 2 14-oz cans of diced tomatoes (or you can use 4 or 5 fresh tomatoes in season OR use the Spaghetti Sauce recipe in the Chapter on Sauces above)
- 1 6-oz can of tomato paste
- 1 cup of water
- 1 medium onion diced
- 2 cloves of garlic minced
- Salt and pepper
- 1 Tbsp oregano
- 1 tsp basil
- 2 Tbsp honey
- 20 – 24 pre-made frozen meatballs

Directions: Place all ingredients except the meatballs in a saucepan and heat to boiling. Using an emersion blender, blend (off the heat) until desired consistency is achieved (the mixture does not need to be pureed; a few small tomato bits are OK). Add the meatballs and simmer for 45 minutes to an hour. Serve over your favorite pasta.
Liver Glycogen Yield per serving (1 ½ cups): **40 – 44 grams** (pasta not included)

Chili

There are dozens of ways to make really great chili. This recipe which serves 4 can be doubled or even tripled and the leftovers frozen. Instead of the ground beef and pork, use chunks of a top round or chuck roast. You can also use green chili peppers (poblano or Serrano for more heat). Sauté them with the onions and garlic.

Ingredients:
- 1 cup diced onion (or two small to medium onions)
- 3-4 cloves garlic, chopped fine
- 2 Tbsp vegetable or olive oil
- 1 pound ground beef, chuck, or veal
- 1 pound ground pork
- 1 Tbsp butter
- 1 can diced or stewed tomatoes (14 ounces)
- 1 can beans (pinto, Great Northern or kidney – your choice) (14 ounces) – no need to drain
- 1 small can (6 ounces) of tomato paste
- 1 cup water (more or less to get desired consistency)
- ¼ cup honey
- 2 Tbsp chili powder (more if desired)
- 1 tsp red chili flakes (more if desired)
- 1 tsp cumin
- 1 tsp ground black pepper
- ½ tsp oregano
- Salt to taste (probably about 1 tsp)

Directions. Sauté the onions and garlic in the oil and butter. Add the ground beef and pork and brown. Add the rest of the ingredients and bring to a boil. Reduce heat and simmer for 30 to 45 minutes or longer while you make the cornbread.

[Note: some of the best champion chili cooks don't bother with sautéing the onions and garlic, or browning the meat. Just put everything into a large pot at once and bring to a boil. Then simmer for 2 to 3 hours. Works for me.]

Liver Glycogen Yield per serving (1 ½ cups): **52 – 54 grams**

[Note: honey.com has a great vegetarian chili recipe using tofu if you are so inclined. It is very similar to the above recipe but without the beef and pork.

Liver Glycogen Yield per serving (1 ½ cup): ~ **30 grams**. The greater **LGY** in chili containing beef and pork versus the vegetarian version is due to the much greater amount of protein (amino acids) found in the 2 pounds of beef and pork than in the 1 pound of tofu. Adding another pound of tofu would only increase the LGY of the vegetarian chili by another 2 – 3 grams per serving.]

From the selected recipes given above, one can easily approximate the amount of liver glycogen produced from a serving of chicken, pork, seafood or beef. Depending on the amount of honey, glazes, sauces or vegetables that accompany the meat, the amount of liver glycogen produced from each average size serving is between **30 and 40 grams** or nearly ½ of the total liver glycogen capacity.

One should note that only about ¾ of the amino acids from protein are available to form liver glycogen. That has been factored into the LGY calculations from all proteins. Furthermore, the length of time from ingestion of most proteins until they are broken down into amino acids and arrive in the liver to form glycogen will vary from 1 to 2 hours or longer. Therefore, proteins are not the best foods to produce an immediate restoration of depleted liver glycogen stores. The honey found in the glazes and sauces in the meat recipes above will, however, produce liver glycogen almost immediately after ingestion.

Chapter 16 - Vegetables and Soups

Roasted vegetables

*P*erhaps one of the most delicious ways to enjoy vegetables is to simply roast them in the oven. During summer months these vegetables can be grilled outdoors in a basket or grilling rack. The options and variations and combinations are end-less. Just for starters here are a few favorites:

- Potatoes
- Sweet potatoes
- Red, yellow, orange or green bell peppers
- Onions, all types as well as green onions
- Whole garlic or garlic cloves
- Turnips
- Parsnips
- Celery root
- Cherry tomatoes (not a vegetable but included here anyway)
- Mushrooms (many varieties)
- Summer squash
- Zucchini
- Butternut or acorn squash or even pumpkin

- Chayote (a mild Mexican squash that looks like a green pear and has a hint of an apple taste)
- Carrots

Directions. Choose your favorites. Cut potatoes, turnips, parsnips, summer squash, zucchini and carrots into similar-sized wedges or rounds so that they will cook in about the same time. Most vegetables can be cooked without peeling. (The celery root needs to be peeled and cubed.) Onions can be quartered or green onions washed, trimmed and cut in 3 to 4 inch lengths. Garlic cloves can be roasted whole as can the cherry tomatoes and small baby carrots.

Place washed and prepared selections on a flat pan with edges (cookie sheet, or large roasting pan) lined with aluminum foil. Drizzle with olive oil and sprinkle liberally with salt and fresh ground pepper. Bake in 375⁰ F oven for 45 minutes or until most vegetables are fork tender. When using cherry tomatoes, you might want to add them to the roasting pan during the last 15 minutes only. Place roasted vegetables on a large serving platter and serve family style. Just before serving, drizzle a small amount of honey over the warm roasted vegetables. Leftover vegetables can be refrigerated and used in soup another day.

Liver Glycogen Yield per serving (1 cup): The range of LGY for most of the vegetables listed above will be between **2 – 8 grams** per cup. A combination of roasted vegetables listed will average **6 – 8 grams** per serving. Even if you consumed 2 cups of vegetables, you would only produce as much liver glycogen from this amount as from 1 tablespoon of honey.

Roasted Vegetable & Chicken Wild Rice Soup
Ingredients:
- 4 cups left-over roasted vegetables
- 4 cups chicken stock
- 1 cup leftover roasted chicken pieces
- 1 cup wild rice
- 1 tsp thyme
- Salt and pepper
- 1 Tbsp honey
- Optional: 1 Tbsp of fresh chopped basil

Directions: Cook the wild rice in 2 cups of the chicken stock. Leave vegetables chunks whole or dice in ½ inch pieces. Place vegetables and cooked rice in two-quart saucepan over medium heat. Add remaining chicken stock, vegetables, and leftover chicken. Season with salt and pepper, thyme or fresh chopped basil. Just before serving add a splash of cream and a tablespoon of honey.

Liver Glycogen Yield per serving (1 ½ cups): **18 – 20 grams**

Roasted Vegetable & Beef Orzo Soup
Ingredients:
- 4 cups left-over roasted vegetables
- 4 cups beef stock
- ½ cup orzo (or ½ cup barley)
- 1 tsp dried oregano or basil
- Salt and pepper

Directions: Add the vegetables, beef stock and ½ cup of orzo to a saucepan. Season with salt and pepper to taste, add fresh chopped basil or oregano. If you prefer, you can thicken the soup with one tablespoon of melted butter mixed with one tablespoon of flour for each two cups of stock.

Liver Glycogen Yield per serving: (1 ½ cups): ~ **6 – 8 grams**

Roasted Squash & Carrot Soup

If you have roasted squash, carrots, sweet potatoes, onions and garlic left over from the roasted vegetables, use these to make this soup. You will need about 4 cups of vegetables total.

Ingredients:
- 1 butternut squash, peeled
- 1 acorn squash, peeled
- 1 sweet potato
- 1 cup carrots
- 3 cups chicken stock or vegetable stock
- ¼ cup honey
- 1 cup cream or half and half
- 1 tsp nutmeg
- Salt and pepper

Directions: Peel and cut the squash, sweet potato and carrots into similar sized pieces. Place on a foil-lined pan or sheet tray. Drizzle with olive oil, and season with salt and pepper. Roast in a 375⁰ F oven for 45 minutes or until fork tender. Place roasted vegetables in a saucepan and add chicken stock. Bring to boil, and then reduce heat to medium. Cook for 20 minutes. Puree the vegetables and stock with an emersion blender or place in blender and puree. Place pureed mix back into the pan and return to medium heat. Add cream or half and half, nutmeg and season to taste with salt and pepper. Keep warm until serving, but do not boil. Serve with a dollop of sour cream and chopped green onions for garnish.

Liver Glycogen Yield per serving (1 ½ cups): **14 – 16 grams**

The reader can see from the few simple vegetable recipes above that the Liver Glycogen Yield from these foods is quite small even with the addition of honey. When a little protein from chicken, beef or half and half is added for example, the LGY jumps up appreciably.

Appendix A lists the approximate LGY for a lot of vegetables that may be included in side dishes or soups. Generally, a vegetable side dish will contribute about **8 – 10 grams** of liver glycogen per serving on the average. This statement is not intended to discourage the consumption of vegetables, for they do provide significant amounts of necessary vitamins and minerals to our diet. When it comes to fueling the brain and restocking the liver glycogen store, however, vegetables rank low on the list behind honey, fruit and proteins from meat and milk products.

Honey.com has recipes for nearly 100 delicious side dishes and soups that use honey. Most will provide the same amount of liver glycogen as the examples above.

Chapter 17 - Desserts

There are so many wonderful dessert recipes that use honey. Honey.com lists over 300 dessert ideas alone. The foodnetwork.com site has hundreds more. In my favorite honey recipe book, *The Buzz on Honey*, Marcella Richman has dozens more including bars, cakes, cookies and other desserts.

So why none in this book? The truth is, desserts are extras. Most desserts are non-essential (except chocolate . . .) Most all dessert recipes that use honey also are loaded with other carbs, flours, fruits, nuts, syrups, oats, chocolate, sugars, cream, butter and shortening. The Liver Glycogen Yield from a serving of most recipes that I have reviewed is small compared to the calorie count. In other words, most deliver more glucose directly to the blood stream (resulting in an elevated blood sugar) than glycogen to the liver.

My advice, enjoy wonderful desserts in moderation as often as you wish. And when possible, opt for those that contain honey. Just don't expect the same healthful benefits from these foods as from those found in the preceding chapters, even though they are made with honey.

"Desserts that contain excessive amounts of glucose to fructose (a higher ratio of fructose to glucose) or foods that contain more than 75 grams of glucose and fructose combined raise blood sugar and store fat."

Remember, the goal is to maximize liver glycogen production with each meal or snack. That is best achieved when foods containing a balance of fructose and glucose, in smaller amounts, or when proteins containing amino acids which form liver glycogen, are consumed. Desserts that contain excessive amounts of glucose to fructose (a higher ratio of glucose to fructose) or foods that contain more than 75 grams of glucose and fructose combined raise blood sugar and store fat.

When consumed regularly and in excess, these foods, though delicious, simply overwhelm the liver's ability to take in and store glycogen. The end result over time is elevated blood sugar which contributes to the development of insulin resistance, and increased risks for all of the diseases and conditions of the metabolic syndrome.

Chapter 18 - Menu Planner

*H*ow shall we then eat? Given the information in the preceding chapters, how do we put it all together in healthy diet planning? While it may not be possible to orchestrate every meal of every day, this final chapter represents suggestions that should help most folks to get on the road to optimum brain fueling. It gives the reader options and calculates estimated Liver Glycogen Yield for each meal.

The Total Liver Glycogen Yield indicated below each menu is a close approximation, at best, of the amount of liver glycogen that may be produced from each meal or snack. The goal is to store enough liver glycogen to get to the next meal. At bedtime, the goal is to ensure enough liver glycogen in the tank to fuel the brain throughout the night fast.

Of course, there will be exceptions. For example, when an excessive amount of sugar or HFCS is ingested from sodas or desserts or snacks, the LGY will be affected, as the liver has to work overtime to metabolize the excess fructose consumed. When that happens, less liver glycogen will be produced and stored. Another exception exists in conditions of advanced insulin resistance. The insulin that is produced is less effective, blood sugar levels remain higher, and less glucose is transported to the brain for fuel. The brain exists in a rather constant state of semi-starvation.

It is not too late to start to take corrective action, and the following menu suggestions just may get you going in the right direction.

Breakfast

Eggs and Bacon
- 2 eggs any style
- 1 strip of bacon
- Fruit cup with honey and yogurt dressing (8 ounces)
- 6 oz orange juice
- 1 slice honey sourdough wheat toast, butter, 1 Tbsp honey
- Coffee or tea, with cream

Total Liver Glycogen Yield per meal: ~ 75 grams

From a liver glycogen perspective, this breakfast ranks as the #1 breakfast combination producing about the same amount of liver glycogen as the liver can store at any one time.

Omelet with Ham, Sausage, Spam or Bacon
- 2 egg omelet with cream cheese, pizza cheese, green onion, mushrooms
- 3 oz of your choice of ham, Spam, sausage, or 2 strips bacon
- 6 oz orange juice
- 1 slice honey sourdough toast
- 1 Tbsp honey
- Coffee or tea

Total Liver Glycogen Yield: 42 – 45 grams

Scrambled eggs and Hawaiian Poke

Poke comes in many varieties in Hawaii. Basically it is some kind of raw fish (usually tuna) cut into small cubes and flavored with any number of seasonings, such as teriyaki, soy sauce, limu (seaweed), sesame oil, sweet chili sauce, chopped green onion, garlic, etc. Salmon will work also. Just lightly sauté the poke in butter or olive oil and serve with scrambled eggs.

- Scrambled eggs
- Poke (3 oz)
- Fruit juice (6 oz)
- English muffin or toast with orange marmalade or jam
- Coffee or tea

Total Liver Glycogen Yield: ~ 35 grams

[Note: by leaving out the honey and using orange marmalade or jam, the total liver glycogen yield is reduced significantly. This breakfast, though it provides plenty of protein, does not immediately act to restock the depleted liver glycogen reserve.]

Oatmeal with fruit

- Oatmeal (1 cup cooked) with 1 Tbsp Honey
- Raisins, dried cranberries or bananas
- Milk (½ cup)
- Fruit juice (6 oz)
- Coffee or tea

Total Liver Glycogen Yield: 39 – 40 grams

[Note: Without the honey, raisins, cranberries or bananas, this breakfast would provide only **17 – 20 grams** of liver glycogen, enough to restock only ¼ of the depleted liver glycogen reserve.]

Granola with fruit

- 1 cup granola
- Your choice of berries, bananas, peaches
- Milk (½ cup)
- Fruit juice (6 oz)
- Coffee or tea

Total Liver Glycogen Yield: 35 – 36 grams

Cereal

Pick your favorite. (We used "heart-healthy" Cheerios in this example and sweetened them with 1 Tbsp of honey just to make the LGY significant.)

- 1 cup Cheerios with 1 Tbsp honey
- Milk (1/2 cup)
- Fruit Juice (6 oz)
- Coffee or Tea

Total Liver Glycogen Yield: ~ 35 grams
[Note: without the honey, this typical American breakfast would provide only **18 – 20 grams** of liver glycogen, even less if juice flavored drinks are used instead of pure juice.]

All ready-to-eat cereals, whether from rice, corn, wheat or other grains are primarily starch (glucose). Most will contain about 3 grams of protein per cup, which will contribute only about 2 grams of liver glycogen per serving. As far as your brain fuel reserve is concerned, eating this typical breakfast is equivalent to starting out on a road trip by placing only 3 – 4 gallons of fuel in the gas tank.

Perhaps an even more "typical" breakfast for many is to grab a cup of coffee and a pastry, donut or piece of toast while rushing out the door. The total Liver Glycogen Yield from this "non-breakfast" is hardly worth mentioning (**2 – 3 grams**).

By adding 1 Tbsp of honey (**17 grams of LGY**), 1 cup of fresh fruit (**10 - 12 grams of LGY**) and 6 - 8 oz of pure fruit juice (~ **8 grams of LGY**), one can boost the total LGY by about 35 grams or nearly half the liver glycogen storage capacity. Even better, why not start the day with some protein from eggs, meat or fish and fill up the tank. Your brain will thank you about midmorning.

Midmorning Snack (10:00 to 10:30 AM)

Fresh fruit
Any kind of fresh seasonal fruit (apples, pears, grapes, bananas, melons, peaches or berries) may be used (total of 1 cup)
Total Liver Glycogen Yield: 10 - 12 grams (avg)
Add 2 Tbsp of yogurt-honey dressing and you will have a LGY of **15 - 18 grams**

Cheese (2 oz) and crackers
Total Liver Glycogen Yield: 3 - 4 grams

Fruit and cheese (1/2 cup fruit and 2 oz Cheese)
Total Liver Glycogen Yield: 8 - 10 grams

Veggies (1 cup) with yogurt and honey dip (2 Tbsp)
Total Liver Glycogen Yield: 10 - 12 grams

Celery, bell peppers, carrots (1 cup) with peanut butter and honey dip (2 Tbsp)
Total Liver Glycogen Yield: 10 - 12 grams

Iced coffee, honey and milk energy drink (16 oz)
Total Liver Glycogen Yield: ~ 30 grams

If breakfast was prior to 7:00 AM, by midmorning, the liver glycogen reserve will be diminished by 30 grams or more depending on one's activity level. The goal is to replenish the liver glycogen store with enough fuel to make it to the next meal.

Lunch (Noon)

Lunches can consist of anything from leftovers to soup and salad to full business lunches to fast food. The examples listed here will give you an idea of the liver glycogen yield possible from a few lunch options.

The temptation to skip lunch as part of an attempt to lose weight should be avoided. By noon, one's brain fuel reserve will be mostly depleted. Intentionally leaving the tank empty forces the brain to initiate fuel conserving and fuel creating mechanisms (*metabolic stress*). The consequences are counter-productive in both the short and long term.

When comparing the total liver glycogen yield, remember that more protein from meats, milk products, and/or fruit in a lunch selection, will produce and store more potential liver glycogen.

Most tossed salads made with a combination of lettuces, vegetables, tomatoes, and cheese sprinkled on top will provide only **5 – 8 grams** of liver glycogen. Add 2 Tbsp of a dressing containing honey and you can boost that amount by **3 – 4 grams**. Add diced chicken or other meats or seafood and the total liver glycogen yield can double to **22 – 26 grams**.

Adding a cup or more of fresh fruit will add another **10 – 15 grams**. Altogether, the goal for lunch should be to consume a combination of foods that will result in the production of **40 – 50 grams** of liver glycogen or enough to fuel the brain until the next meal.

Soup and sandwich

Sliced luncheon meats, cheeses, lettuce, tomato, pickles (your choice), and a little mayonnaise with 2 slices of honey sourdough bread
Roasted squash and carrot soup
Total Liver Glycogen Yield: 22 - 25 grams

Chicken salad with toast or English muffin

Chicken salad with celery, grapes, walnuts and mayonnaise, lettuce
Total Liver Glycogen Yield: ~ 20 grams
[Note: add 1 Tbsp of honey to the chicken salad and you can increase the LGY to **24 grams**]

Tortilla roll-up with cream cheese spread and honey

1 large flour tortilla with cream cheese spread, thinly sliced meats or meat pate, cheese, cucumbers
Total Liver Glycogen Yield: 10 - 12 grams
Add a cup of soup for an additional **8 - 10 grams**

Soup and Salad

Chicken and wild rice soup
Tossed salad with honey mustard dressing
Total Liver Glycogen Yield: 28 - 30 grams

Chilidog and honey-lemonade

Hot dog and bun with chili and cheese
12 oz honey-lemonade
Total Liver Glycogen Yield: 18 - 20 grams

Cheeseburger and French fries with 16 oz soft drink

Total Liver Glycogen Yield: 24 - 25 grams
[Note: while the LGY from the hamburger patty and cheese will produce some liver glycogen, the 40+ grams of sucrose or HFCS from the soft drink

will not produce any significant amount. The net effect will be an elevated blood sugar for 1 to 2 hours followed by a drop in blood sugar that will only result in more appetite hormone release. And with only 1/3 of the liver glycogen tank being filed up with this lunch, there probably won't be enough fuel for the brain to make it to dinner.]

Grilled Cheese and Tomato Bisque Soup
   Thick sliced crusty bread, provolone cheese with pickled cauliflower, red peppers and honey relish
   Tomato Bisque soup (recipe on page 185)
   Total Liver Glycogen Yield: 22 – 25 grams

Afternoon Snack (3:00 PM)

The same snack items listed in the midmorning snack section on page 223 can be repeated during the afternoon. The goal should be to consume food combinations that provide **20 to 30 grams** of liver glycogen yield or enough to fuel the brain until the dinner hour.

Evening Meal (around 6:00 PM)

The options for dinner are virtually endless. The goal for this meal is to produce enough liver glycogen to fill up the tank in preparation for the night fast. The best way to do this is with a combination of proteins, fruits and vegetables that provide both immediate and delayed liver glycogen formation. Remember, fruits and some vegetables will result in rather immediate liver glycogen formation; proteins (or amino acids) will be available to form liver glycogen in 2 – 3 hours. If you eat around 6:00 PM your brain fuel tank will be full around 8:00 to 9:00 PM. *Eating later in the evening is not unhealthy.* In fact, eating later only ensures that the liver glycogen reserve will be full closer to bedtime.

Several menu options are presented just to give you an idea of the possible liver glycogen yield from each combination. Using the liver glycogen yield from each food item (as found in **Appendix A**), one can choose and substitute according to your family's tastes. Recipes can be found in the preceding chapters or in the other references listed. The majority of liver glycogen will be produced from the protein selections as well as those menus that have fruit and/or honey in the sauces or glazes.

Serving size for each entry has been intentionally left out. Portion control is an essential aspect of weight loss so if that is your goal, limit the portion sizes of protein to 3 – 4 oz, the vegetables or pasta to about 1 cup or less and the fruit to about 1 cup. Larger portions will also have a greater liver glycogen yield.

Salmon Filet with Honey Lemon Cream Sauce
Steamed broccoli with cheese sauce
Fruit platter (strawberries, green grapes, bananas, melon)
Liver Glycogen Yield per meal: ~ 40 grams

Tilapia filet with Mango Salsa (recipe on pages 205 and 188)
Steamed rice
Mango salsa
Steamed cauliflower
Liver Glycogen Yield per meal: ~ 28 grams

Crockpot Honey Sesame Chicken
Steamed rice
Slaw with honey, balsamic vinegar dressing

Liver Glycogen Yield per meal: ~ 60 grams

Crockpot Honey Pork Roast
  Roasted vegetables
  Fruit Salad with Honey and Yogurt Dressing
  Total Liver Glycogen Yield per meal: ~ 65 grams

Spaghetti and Meatballs
  Pasta
  Tossed salad with honey mustard dressing
  Total Liver Glycogen Yield per meal: ~ 50 grams

Grilled Chicken with Honey Orange Glaze
  Steamed vegetables (your choice)
  Fresh fruit (melon, berries) and cheese platter
  Total Liver Glycogen Yield per meal: ~ 50 grams

Honey Lime Chicken Enchiladas (recipe on page 201)
  Refried beans
  Fresh salsa
  Shredded lettuce and diced tomato for garnish
  Total Liver Glycogen Yield per meal: ~ 45 grams

Meatloaf with Honey and Pine nuts (recipe on page 205)
  Mashed potatoes with garlic
  Green beans and pearl onions
  Total Liver Glycogen Yield per meal: ~ 30 grams

Chili with Cornbread and Honey
  Recipes can be found on pages 207 and 196.
  Total Liver Glycogen Yield per meal: ~ 75 grams

Bedtime Snack (10:30 to 11:00 PM)

1 – 2 Tbsp of unfiltered honey
Total Liver Glycogen Yield: 15 – 30 grams

Of course there are other snacks that can be eaten at bedtime. The important thing is to avoid foods that will take a long time to digest (proteins and milk products) and juices that contain up to 80% water. All are good, yet the digestive track is powering down during sleep and the digestive processes are slowed significantly, making absorption much slower.

Honey is the "gold-standard" food for consumption just before sleep. It is rapidly absorbed from the digestive tract and turned into liver glycogen within minutes. The glucose component of honey triggers a small insulin release that starts the HYMN cycle resulting in sleep. The liver glycogen produced from honey tops off the liver glycogen reserve ensuring enough brain fuel to get through the night without interruption, thus promoting recovery physiology to take place during rest.

Putting It All Together

Most of you have picked up on the basics that underlie meal planning in this chapter. Just in case you need reinforcement, the following summary of foods to include and foods to avoid will wrap it all up.

It really is not necessary to count calories or avoid fats as much as it is about feeding your brain first. It may seem counter-intuitive, but our brains really can starve in spite of our excess consumption. What's important is consuming the right balance of fructose and glucose along with an appropriate amount of amino acids with every meal or snack so that our liver glycogen reserves can be filled up or topped off.

Portion control and moderation are also important factors to consider. As you may have noted, 3 – 4 ounces of meat or fish with every meal is sufficient to produce about **25 – 35 grams** of liver glycogen from amino acids. A cup of fruit with a honey yogurt sauce will add another **20 – 25 grams**. A serving of vegetables does not add much to the liver glycogen total. The important thing to remember with vegetables is to limit the ones that are mainly starch (glucose) such as white potatoes, rice, and pastas.

Foods to include that supply brain fuel:
- Honey
- Raisins, dates, figs
- Fresh fruit
- Pure fruit juices
- Any green or leafy vegetables
- Other yellow, red or non-white vegetables
- Homemade sauces and salad dressings made with honey
- Whole milk products, yogurt and sour cream
- Cheeses of all kinds
- Eggs
- Meat, poultry, fish

Foods to limit or avoid:
- Sugar, syrups
- Artificial sweeteners
- Low-fat or "diet" foods that contain sugar or HFCS or artificial sweeteners
- Canned fruit in syrup
- Canned or bottled sauces
- White potatoes

- Potato chips
- White rice
- Pastas
- White bread
- Breakfast cereals of all kinds
- Juice flavored drinks
- Soda
- Processed foods
- Bottled salad dressings with added sugar, HFCS
- Baked goods that are high in white flour and sugar

The primary reason to avoid or limit the foods in the group above is less about calories or carbs. The reason to avoid them is that they do not contribute significantly to the brain fuel reserve. They do not form liver glycogen. In fact, when eaten regularly and in excessive amounts, they actually deplete the liver glycogen reserve and produce a degree of chronic brain starvation with both short- and long-term health consequences.

Feed your brain first. A brain that is well fueled means better health for the body, improved sleep and better aging. It is never too late to start.

Glenn's Story – A Happy Ending

G lenn was just a few days past his 77th birthday when he handed me an envelope. Inside were three pages of lab results from his recent physical exam and four pages from his physical exam exactly one year ago. His smile gave indication that something good was about to be revealed.

Several months before, I had shared with Glenn and his wife Sandy, the principles of brain fueling – eat foods that have a balance of fructose and glucose in order to produce more liver glycogen; don't go to bed hungry; limit the consumption of starchy, glucose-rich foods; consume more honey, especially at bedtime and in the morning.

Glenn had reason to be concerned. He was a pilot and though his flying now was limited to occasional trips in his twin engine Cessna, he subjected himself to the mandatory annual flight physicals required of someone his age. A year ago, his lab work revealed an elevated cholesterol level (237 mg/dL – normal being below 199 mg/dL) with the LDL-cholesterol fraction markedly elevated (162 mg/dL – normal being below 99 mg/dL). His triglycerides were normal but at the upper limit of the normal range. His doctor had recommend lipid lowering drugs, which Glenn had taken for a while, but later abandoned due to the unpleasant side effects.

A few weeks before his scheduled flight physical, Glenn had asked if I thought honey would help with his cholesterol lab values. My answer was an unqualified yes.

A few days before his appointment, Glenn checked with me again, this time to ask how honey might affect his fasting blood sugar. My response was to indicate that fasting blood sugar readings are typically elevated due to what is known as the "dawn phenomenon." The brain, sensing that its fuel supply is low or depleted after several hours of fasting (such as overnight), initiates adrenal-driven stress resulting in new glucose being formed from amino acids. Thus the blood sugar reading after an overnight fast is always going to be artificially elevated.

My suggestion to Glenn was to have his tablespoon of honey at bedtime and again in the morning an hour or so before his blood samples were to be drawn. Though this advice might seem counter-intuitive to some, and contrary to his doctor's instructions regarding fasting, Glenn did as I suggested.

The results were in. The envelope opened. Now it was my turn to smile. Glenn's total cholesterol was 175 mg/dL, down from 237 mg/dL, a drop of 62 mg/dL. His LDL-cholesterol was down from 162 mg/dL to 113 mg/dL, and though still slightly elevated, not something that warranted intervention. In addition, Glenn's VLDL (Very Low Density Lipoprotein) was down from 26 mg/dL to 14 mg/dL. Though neither value was elevated, the drop was significant.

Even more remarkable was his triglyceride level. A year ago, Glenn's triglycerides were 131 mg/dL. This year they were 69 mg/dL, a drop of 62 mg/dL. While both readings were within the "normal range," this dramatic reduction was further indication of the therapeutic effects of adding regular "doses" of honey to one's diet.

An understanding of the metabolism of honey as detailed throughout this book would indicate that Glenn's dramatic results should not be viewed with surprise. Yet, Glenn's physician remained unconvinced.

The same can be said for a majority of physicians today who practice by the numbers, and "treat the numbers" with a host of costly prescription drugs that, while they may bring the numbers down, do nothing for the underlying cause of one's condition.

Is Glenn's metabolic response to consuming honey typical? Is this something that can be expected by everyone? Although the research confirmation so far comes from limited animal and human studies, much anecdotal evidence is being accumulated that would answer these questions affirmatively. Dozens of folks have written to me and shared similar results.

Unfortunately, it will take years for long-term population studies to be completed if they were to be considered. The economic reality is that honey is a "medicine without profit."[69] There are over 300 varietals of honey in the U.S. and Canada and no clinical research director would consider an intervention study with this many variables. No pharmaceutical company would fund such a study, which would no doubt show significantly better results from a natural food than from costly drugs, at least when it comes to cholesterol, triglyceride and blood sugar control.

The good news is that one does not need to wait to join *The Honey Revolution*. There are no risks, side effects or negative health consequences from starting today. You may not have the dramatic results that Glenn did in such a short time, but it is quite likely that you will experience better health and reduced risks of suffering the consequences of all the metabolic conditions discussed in this book.

In the Old Testament book of Deuteronomy, Moses gives us an expansive song citing God's abundant nutritional provisions for the children of Israel. Receive his words as a closing Good Word to you:

*"He made then ride over the highlands; he let them feast on the crops of the fields. He nourished them with **honey** from the cliffs, with olive oil from the hard rock."* (Deuteronomy 32:13, New Living Translation)

May you also experience these blessings.

Appendix A

Table of Estimated Liver Glycogen Yield (LGY) per Serving of Common Foods in Grams (Values rounded to the nearest 0.1-gram) [G = glucose; F = fructose; S = sucrose] *

*Glucose, fructose and sucrose amounts for these selected foods have been taken from nutritiondata. com, USDA SR-21 and other publicly available sources. The calculation of the estimated liver glycogen yield is the sole responsibility of the author. For an example of how LGY is calculated see **Appendix B**.

Food Item	Serving Size	G	F	S	LGY
Honey	1 Tbsp	7.5	8.6	0	17
Fruit					
Apple	1 cup	3	7.4	2.6	12
Applesauce	1 cup	5.6	14.3	2.8	22
Apricots	1 cup	3.7	1.5	9.1	11
Avocados	1 cup	0.7	0.2	0.1	2.8
Bananas	1 cup	23.3	10.9	5.4	17.6

Bananas	1 cup	23.3	10.9	5.4	17.6
Blackberries	1 cup	3.3	3.5	0.1	6.5
Blueberries	1 cup	7.2	7.4	0.2	14
Cherries	1 cup	10.1	8.3	0.2	20
Clementines	1 fruit	1.2	1.2	4.4	5
Cranberries	1 cup	3.6	0.7	0.1	1.1
Dates	1/4 cup	7.3	7.3	9	20
Grapefruit	1 cup	3.7	4.1	8.1	13
Grapes, seedless	1 cup	10.8	12.3	0.8	24
Kiwi	1 cup	7.3	7.7	0.3	16.9
Melon, honeydew	1 cup	4.7	5.2	4.4	12
Melon, cantaloupe	1 cup	2.7	3.3	7.7	11
Nectarines	1 cup	2.2	2	7	8.6
Oranges, naval	1 cup	3.3	3.7	7	11.5
Orange juice	1 cup	5.8	6.4	8.7	17.6
Olives, green	½ cup	0.5	0.5	0.2	2-3
Olives, ripe	½ cup	1	1	0.4	3-4
Peaches	1 cup	3	2.4	7.3	10
Pear	1 cup	4.4	10	1.3	15.5
Pineapple	1 cup	2.9	3.5	9.9	12
Plums	1 cup	8.4	5	2.6	12
Raisins, seedless	1/4 cup	13.4	12	0.2	22
Raspberries	1 cup	2.3	2.9	0.2	6
Strawberries	1 cup	3	3.7	0.7	8.5
Tangerines	1 cup	4.1	4.7	11.8	16
Tomatoes	1 cup	2.3	2.5	0	5.7
Tomato juice	1 cup	3.3	3.7	0.6	8.5
Watermelon	1 cup	2.4	5.2	1.9	9
Vegetables					
Artichokes	1 cup	0.4	0	1.2	3.6
Asparagus	1 cup	0.7	1.4	0.1	1.5

Beans, green	1 cup	1.1	1.3	0.3	4
Beans, kidney	1 cup	23	0	4.7	8.5
Beans, navy	1 cup	68.8	0	6.9	33.6
Beans, pinto	1 cup	25.9	0	0.5	10.4
Bell pepper, green	1 cup	1.7	1.7	0.2	4.3
Bell pepper, red	1 cup	2.9	3.4	0	7.2
Broccoli	1 cup	0.8	1.2	0.1	4.4
Brussels sprouts	1 cup	0.7	0.8	0.4	3.6
Cabbage	1 cup	1.5	1.3	0.1	3.5
Cabbage, red	1 cup	1.5	1.3	0.5	4
Carrots	1 cup	2.6	0.7	4.6	3.7
Cauliflower	1 cup	1.3	0	0	< 1
Celery	1 cup	0.6	0.5	0.1	2
Corn	1 cup	25.9	0.7	3.1	5.2
Cucumber	1/2 cup	0.8	1	0	2.4
Lettuce, iceberg	1 cup	0.7	0.7	0	1.8
Lettuce, romaine	1 cup	0.2	0.4	0	0.9
Lettuce, butter head	1 cup	0.2	0.3	0	1
Mushrooms, white	1 cup	1	0.1	0	2.5
Oatmeal, cooked	1 cup	27	0	0.6	3.5
Okra	1 cup	0.4	0.2	0.4	2.1
Onions	1 cup	3.2	2	1.6	7.1
Pasta	100 gm	25	0	0	3
Peas	1 cup	0.2	0.6	7.2	9.6
Potatoes, baked	1 cup	26	0.5	0.6	3.7
Potatoes, French fried - vegetable oil	1 cup	34	0	0.2	3
Potatoes, mashed (from dehydrated flakes)	1 cup	43	0.6	0.6	4.8

Radishes	1 cup	1.2	0.8	0.1	2.6
Rice, white	1 cup	35	0	0.1	2.6
Rice, brown long grain	1 cup	41	0	0.7	3
Soy (edamame)	1 cup	0	0.2	1.7	12
Squash, summer	1 cup	0.8	1.1	0	2.8
Sweet potatoes	1 cup	18.1	0.9	4.7	8
Turnips	1 cup	54	0.4	0.4	1.9
Turnip greens	1 cup	0.3	0.2	0	1
Zucchini	1 cup	0.9	1.2	0	3
Nuts and Seeds					
Almonds	1 cup	1.2	0.1	5.1	22.3
Brazil nuts	1 cup	0.3	0	3.1	13.6
Cashew nuts	1 cup	32	0.05	5.8	16.3
Hazelnuts / filberts	1 cup	0.7	0.1	4.8	14
Macadamia nuts	1 cup	1.5	0.1	5.3	9.4
Pecans	1 cup	0.5	0	4.3	8.5
Pistachio nuts	1 cup	2.7	0.2	8.6	21
Walnuts	1 cup	0.2	0.1	2.8	13
Flaxseed	1 cup	0.7	0	1.9	20.5
Peanut butter	1 cup	22.4	0	6.2	39
Seafood and Shellfish					
Food Item	**Serving Size**	**Amount Protein**	**Available Amino Acids**		**LGY**
Crab, Dungeness	3 oz	19	14		12
Crayfish	3 oz	14.3	10.7		9
Lobster	3 oz	17.4	13		11
Shrimp	3 oz	17.8	13.4		11
Bass	3 oz	20.6	15.5		13
Catfish	3 oz	15.9	11.9		10

Cod	3 oz	19.4	14.6	12
Halibut	3 oz	22.7	17	15
Perch	3 oz	21.1	15.8	14
Salmon	3 oz	21.6	16.2	14
Snapper	3 oz	22.4	16.8	15
Trout	3 oz	22.6	17	15
Tuna, fresh	3 oz	25.4	19	17
Clams	3 oz	21.7	16.3	14
Oysters	3 oz	8	6	5
Meat and Poultry				
Food Item	Serving Size	Amount Protein	Available Amino Acid	LGY
Chicken, roasted	1 cup	37.8	28.4	23
Beef, roasted	4 oz	25-35	19-26	~ 18
Hamburger	3 oz	21.5	16.1	13
Bacon	2 slices	6	4.5	3
Canadian Bacon	2 slices	11.4	8.55	7
Ham, cured	3 oz	23.1	17.3	15
Pork tenderloin	3 oz	18.3	13.7	12
Pork, ground	3 oz	21.8	16.35	14
Pulled pork	1 cup	34.2	25.65	21
Pork chop	7 oz	41.2	30.9	24
Bison, roasted	3 oz	28.7	21.5	17
Leg of lamb	3 oz	23.2	17.4	14
Veal, braised	3 oz	22	16.5	13
Veal, ground	3 oz	20.7	15.5	12
Processed Meats / Luncheon Meats				
Beef bologna	1 slice	3.3	2.5	2
Beef pastrami	1 slice	6.1	4.6	3.5

Beef sausage	1 oz	5.1	3.8	3
Pork bologna	1 slice	4.3	3.2	2.6
Turkey bologna	1 slice	3.2	2.4	2
Bratwurst	2.33 oz	8.1	6	5
Chicken breast	2 slices 42 g	7.1	5.3	4
Spam	2 oz	7.5	5.6	4.5
Processed Meats / Luncheon Meats				
Frankfurter, beef	1 (52g)	6	4.5	3.6
Frankfurter, beef and pork	1 (45g)	5.2	3.9	3.1
Frankfurter, chicken	1 (45g)	7	5.25	4
Ham, canned	1 oz (28g)	4.5	3.4	2.5
Luncheon meat, beef	1 oz (28g)	5	3.75	3
Olive loaf	1 oz (28g)	2.8	2.1	1.6
Salami	27 g	5.6	4.2	3.4
Little smokies	57 g	7.1	5.3	4.2
Pepperoni	28 g	6.4	4.8	3.9

Dairy Products and Eggs ***
(Values rounded to nearest 0.01 gram)
[G = Glucose; F = Fructose; S = Sucrose; L = Lactose;
AAA = Available Amino Acids
Each ~ indicates missing or incomplete value]

Milk and Dairy Products							
Food Item	Size	G	F	S	L	AAA	LGY
Butter	1 cup	0	0	0	0.1	1.9	2
Butter-milk	1 cup	0	0	0	11	4.9	14
Mayo-nnaise	1 cup	40	0	15	0	2.1	3
Whole Milk	1 cup	0	0	0	12.8	5.9	16
Milk, 2%	1 cup	0.02	0.02	0.02	12.7	6	16

Milk, 1%	1 cup	0	0	0	12.7	6	16
Milk, evap	½ cup	~	~	~	12.7	6.45	18
Half & Half	1 cup	~	~	~	10.4	5.4	14
Heavy Cream	1 cup	~	~	~	0.3	3.7	3
Cottage cheese	1 cup	0	0	0	6	18.8	22
Sour cream	1 cup	0	0	0	8.1	3.6	11
Yogurt	1 cup	~	~	~	11.4	6.4	16
Cheeses							
Mozza-rella	1 cup	0.6	0.2	0.1	0.1	18.6	16
Cheddar	1 cup	~	~	0.3	0.3	24.7	19
Feta	1 cup	~	~	~	6.1	21.3	22
Cream cheese	1 cup	0	0	0	7.4	10.4	16
Blue	1 cup	~	~	~	0.7	21.7	18
Eggs							
Eggs ****	2	0.2	0.1	0.1	0.15	10.2	10.2

[Notes and Assumptions: **Liver Glycogen Yield** calculations. As we have said earlier in the book, there is no easy or noninvasive way to accurately determine the amount of glycogen that may be present in the liver at any given time. Nor is there an absolute way of determining the amount of liver glycogen that might result from the ingestion of a particular food.

Here is what we do know. Fructose and glucose when ingested together in nearly equal amounts form liver glycogen directly. Fructose reaches the liver first, aided by dual transport mechanisms in the intestinal wall that transport it into the blood stream. When it reaches the liver, fructose "unlocks" glucokinase from the liver cell nucleus that then allows glucose to be brought into the liver to form glycogen. Fructose is also converted directly to glycogen in the liver by the simple process of phosphorylation (adding a phosphate ion to the fructose on one end of the 6-carbon chain). Without fructose, glucose simply passes through the liver and into the general circulation, raising insulin levels that drive most of the glucose into the muscle and fat cells.

It is reasonable to conclude that most fructose and glucose ingested together in equal ratio at any given time is immediately converted to liver glycogen. For example, if one tablespoon (21 grams) of honey containing 7.5 and 8.6 grams of glucose and fructose respectively is ingested, approximately 15 grams of liver glycogen will be produced. Some glucose will remain in the blood and result in a small controlled insulin release. This glucose will be transported into the muscle and fat cells under the influence of insulin and thus not form liver glycogen.

Our calculations of liver glycogen yield tend to err on the low side for foods containing high levels of starch (glucose) or complex carbohydrates that are converted to glucose. Glucose from these sources actually ends up in muscle or fat cells due to the rapid action of insulin that is released as blood glucose rises. Foods containing a greater proportion of glucose (or starch) compared to fructose, such as a mixed carbohydrate meal or some fruit such as bananas with more than twice as much glucose than fructose, will also result in less glycogen formation, again due to the action of insulin. A lesser amount of liver glycogen will be formed due to the rapid action of insulin driving glucose from the blood into the cells.

Some foods, especially fruits, citrus juices or carrots, contain additional amounts of sucrose (glucose and fructose combined in a single molecule). Enzymes in the body rapidly separate the glucose from the fructose into separate molecules. Total liver glycogen yield for these foods has been adjusted upward to allow for the equal additional glucose and fructose. Foods with larger amounts of sucrose, however, typically raise insulin levels faster, triggering a higher release of insulin which results in the glucose portion being driven into the muscle and fat cells where is not available for liver glycogen formation. The total LGY is decreased by 10 to 20% for these high sucrose-containing foods to allow for this "sucrose anomaly."

Many vegetables such as beans or potatoes contain little or no fructose. Values given for total glucose include the large amounts of starch that each contain, as starch is glucose.

Fruits and vegetables also contain some protein (not shown in the tables above). Amino acids from these proteins do contribute to the production of some liver glycogen and that has been factored in.

When more than 75 to 80 grams of combined fructose and glucose are ingested at any one time, no new liver glycogen can be formed as the liver's storage capacity is exceeded. At that point, the liver stops forming glycogen and acts immediately to metabolize the excess fructose into trioses that form triglycerides. The excess glucose is returned to the blood where insulin works to drive it into the cells where it is stored as fat. The same is true for foods containing a large amount of sucrose. Glucose from starchy foods or other carbohydrates that do not contain much fructose do not contribute to liver glycogen formation directly. This glucose also raises insulin levels that force the glucose into the muscle and fat cells where it is stored as fat.

Foods containing amino acids from protein (nuts, seeds, meats and fish also produce liver glycogen even though they contain no fructose. Approximately 75% of the amino acids from protein can be used by the liver and converted to liver glycogen. The total LGY for all meats and poultry have been reduced by 15 to 20% to account for some transfer from the blood to the brain cells and other tissues for direct use. The estimated amount of liver glycogen yield reflects the amount of amino acids present in these foods. Amino acids from protein consumed during a mixed meal will not form liver glycogen as rapidly as fructose/glucose containing foods. The time required for digestion of proteins into amino acids is considerably longer.

** The higher than expected LGY from nuts comes from the protein and amino acid content of these foods.

*** Milk and dairy products. Milk and dairy products contain lactose or "milk sugar" as well as other sugars. Lactose is a disaccharide that is rapidly digested into glucose and galactose. Galactose, like fructose, is metabolized in the liver and facilitates the formation of liver glycogen just as fructose does. Milk and dairy products also contain protein and amino acids that contribute to the formation of liver glycogen. The estimated LGY from milk and dairy products is arrived at by combining the amount of glycogen produced from lactose, other sugars, as well as the available amino acids from protein.

**** Eggs contain a small amount of sucrose, lactose, maltose and galactose that contribute, along with amino acids, to glycogen formation.]

Appendix B

Example: Calculation of Liver Glycogen Yield per Serving of Homemade Catsup

Food Item	Amount	Wt/Vol	Fructose	Glucose
Tomatoes*	3 cups	24 oz	7.5 gm	6.75 gm
Onion*	1/2 cup	4 oz	2.4 gm	2 gm
Tomato Paste*	3/4 cup	6 oz	12 gm	11.7 gm
Vinegar	1/2 cup	4 oz	< 0.1 gm	< 0.1 gm
Honey	3/4 cup	6 oz	103 gm	90 gm
Salt	1 tsp			
Onion Powder	1/2 tsp		< 0.5 gm	< 0.5 gm
Garlic Powder	1/2 tsp		< 0.5 gm	< 0.5 gm
Totals	4 cups	32 oz	~126 gm	~128 gm
Total Liver Glycogen Possible from All Ingredients Combined				~250 gm
Serving Size				2 Tbsp
Estimated Glycogen Yield per Serving				~ 8 gm

*These items contain a small amount of sucrose as well as fructose and glucose. Since sucrose is equal parts glucose and fructose, the total amount of glucose and fructose has been adjusted up to account for this. For calculations of liver glycogen yields from other foods, compared to honey – the gold standard for liver glycogen formation. See the **Table of Estimated Liver Glycogen Yield for Common Foods in Grams, Appendix A.**

Appendix C

INTERNATIONAL TABLE OF GLYCEMIC INDEX
(GI) AND GLYCEMIC LOAD (GL) [71]

[Note: Selected foods and values have been taken from the full table as published in *American Journal of Clinical Nutrition,* 2002. The complete table can be found in the *Am J Clin Nutr* 2002; 76: 5–56. Printed in USA. © 2002 American Society for Clinical Nutrition.]

* Where more than one food in each food type were listed, the mean of the values is given as the first value. Note the wide disparity in the range of values for GI depending on which reference standard, glucose = 100 (the first value) or white bread = 100 (the second value), was used in the calculations.

Food Category / Item	GI*	Serving Size (g)	Available Carbs (g)	GL
Bakery Goods				
Cake doughnut	76-108	47	23	17
Croissant	67-96	57	26	17
Bran Muffin	60-85	57	24	15
Pancakes	67-96	80	58	39
Waffles	76-109	35	13	10
Scones	92-131	25	9	7
Beverages				
Coca Cola	63	8.5 oz (250 ml)	26	16
Apple Juice	40-57	8.5 oz	29	12
Cranberry Juice	52-80	8.5 oz	31	16
Grapefruit Juice	48-69	8.5 oz	22	11
Orange Juice	50-71	8.5 oz	26	13
Pineapple Juice	46-66	8.5 oz	34	16
Tomato Juice	38-54	8.5 oz	9	4
Gatorade	78-111	8.5 oz	15	12
Breads				
Bagel	72-103	70	35	25
Oat-bran	47-68	30	18	9
Whole-wheat	53-76	30	20	11
White-enriched	71-101	30	13	9
Cereals				
All-Bran (Kellogg's)	38-54	30	23	9
Bran Flakes (Kellogg's)	74-106	30	18	13
Cheerios (General Mills)	74-106	30	20	15
Cornflakes (Kellogg's)	81-116	30	26	21

Froot Loops (Kellogg's)	69-98	30	26	18
Grape Nuts (Kraft Foods)	71-102	30	21	15
Raisin Bran (Kellogg's)	61-87	30	19	12
Rice Krispies (Kellogg's)	82-117	30	26	22
Shredded Wheat	75-107	30	20	15
Special K (Kellogg's)	69-98	30	21	14

Appendix D

The Neuro-degenerative Process Summarized

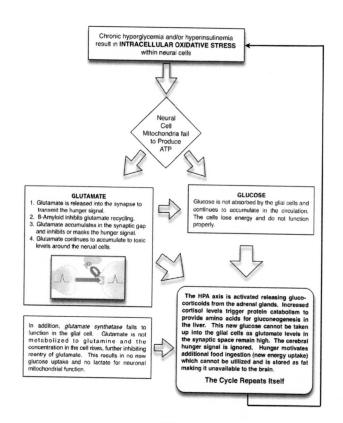

Chronic hyperglycemia and/or hyperinsulinemia result in **INTRACELLULAR OXIDATIVE STRESS** within neural cells

Neural Cell Mitochondria fail to Produce ATP

GLUTAMATE
1. Glutamate is released into the synapse to transmit the hunger signal.
2. β-Amyloid inhibits glutamate recycling.
3. Glutamate accumulates in the synaptic gap and inhibits or masks the hunger signal.
4. Glutamate continues to accumulate to toxic levels around the nerual cells.

GLUCOSE
Glucose is not absorbed by the glial cells and continues to accumulate in the circulation. The cells lose energy and do not function properly.

In addition, *glutamate synthetase* fails to function in the glial cell. Glutamate is not metabolized to glutamine and the concentration in the cell rises, further inhibiting reentry of glutamate. This results in no new glucose uptake and no lactate for neuronal mitochondrial function.

The HPA axis is activated releasing gluco-corticoids from the adrenal glands. Increased cortisol levels trigger protein catabolism to provide amino acids for gluconeogenesis in the liver. This new glucose cannot be taken up into the glial cells as glutamate levels in the synaptic space remain high. The cerebral hunger signal is ignored. Hunger motivates additional food ingestion (new energy uptake) which cannot be utilized and is stored as fat making it unavailable to the brain.

The Cycle Repeats Itself

Endnotes

Acknowledgements

[1] *The Honey Revolution – Restoring the Health of Future Generations* and *The Honey Revolution – Abridged,* Ronald E Fessenden, MD, MPH and Mike McInnes, MRPS, WorldClassEmprise, LLC, 2008, 2010

Foreword

[2] Lactose is a disaccharide made up of galactose and fructose. Galactose, like fructose, is primarily metabolized in the liver where it is stored as glucose. Galactose also facilitates the incorporation of glucose into the liver, taking glucose out of the blood and storing it there. Thus both lactose from milk and glucose and fructose from honey serve similar purposes in human metabolism by storing fuel for the brain.

Introduction

[3] Blood glucose levels are maintained in the body within a fairly narrow range under most circumstances. That range is 70 to 110 mg/dL.

[4] Glycogen phosphorylase breaks up glycogen in the liver into individual glycogen molecules so that they can be released back into the blood.

[5] Work by a Montreal team led by Professor Marc Lavoie has demonstrated that IGFBP-1 is the signal that warns the brain of a depleting liver glycogen level. It works in inverse proportion to the actual liver glycogen status. When liver glycogen levels are high, IGFBP-1 is low. When liver glycogen levels are low, IGFBP-1 is elevated.

Chapter 1

[6] Glial cells are endothelial cells that make up the blood-brain barrier and provide metabolic support for the neurons or brain cells.

[7] Gluconeogenesis is the process by which "new glucose" is formed from amino acids in the liver. The brain orchestrates this process by initiating the release of adrenalin and cortisol from the adrenal glands. These hormones facilitate the conversion of protein from muscle cells into amino acids, which are then carried back to the liver where new glucose is formed.

[8] This system is known as the hypothalamus/pituitary/adrenal or HPA axis. It includes the hypothalamus and pituitary portions of the brain as well as the adrenal glands located near the kidneys.

Tom's Story

[9] It is well documented in previous books in *The Honey Revolution* series that excessive consumption of HFCS

contributes to the production of triglycerides that when stored in the liver result in what pathologists call a "fatty liver."

[10] *Chronic partial nocturnal starvation* is repeated brain starvation that occurs nightly when the liver glycogen reserve becomes depleted during sleep. *Chronic partial sleep loss* occurs as a result of brain starvation that triggers the release of adrenalin and cortisol resulting in interrupted and short sleep. *Chronic intermittent metabolic stress* is associated with adrenalin and cortisol release. It is a protective mechanism initiated by the brain to provide fuel for itself when liver glycogen reserves are depleted.

Chapter 2

[11] HbA1c (hemoglobin A1c) or glycated hemoglobin is a form of hemoglobin to which glucose molecules become attached. HbA1c is used to identify the average blood glucose concentration over a period of weeks prior to the time the lab test is taken. A normal HbA1c measurement is considered to be $\leq 6.5\%$.

[12] The normal range for blood glucose (blood sugar) in the human is considered to be between 70 and 110 mg/dL or approximately 4 - 6 mmol/L.

[13] It is the hormones of the adrenal gland, cortisol and adrenaline, which are primarily responsible for the metabolic stress that results in the conditions and diseases of the metabolic syndrome.

[14] The Institute of Medicine recommends that American and Canadian adults get between 45-65% of dietary

energy requirements from carbohydrates. Food and Nutrition Board (2002/2005). "Dietary Reference Intakes for Energy, Carbohydrate, Fiber, Fat, Fatty Acids, Cholesterol, Protein, and Amino Acids." Washington, DC: *The National Academies Press*, page 769

[15] The World Health Organization (WHO) sets the range for total carbohydrates at 55-75% and 10% from simple sugars, from the Joint WHO/FAO expert consultation (2003). "Diet, Nutrition and the Prevention of Chronic Diseases" (PDF) Geneva: World Health Organization, pp. 55-56

[16] "The Corn Refiners Association (CRA) in September 2010 petitioned the Food and Drug Administration (FDA) asking it to allow the term 'corn sugar' as an alternative label declaration for high fructose corn syrup (HFCS). HFCS has suffered from a spate of bad publicity in recent years, and food and beverage manufacturers have been increasingly switching it out of their products in preference for beet or cane sugar (sucrose).

The CRA has said that the reason it filed a petition with the FDA was to be clear with consumers about what HFCS is: A sugar made from corn. The CRA – a trade association that represents the corn refining industry in the United States – has repeatedly stressed that HFCS is not high in fructose, even though that is what the name may suggest. In fact it contains proportions of fructose and glucose that are similar to sucrose.

President of the Corn Refiners Association, Audrae Erickson, told FoodNavigator-USA.com: "The words 'high fructose corn syrup' have caused confusion . . . This is all about consumer clarity on the ingredient label." She said that in much the same way that there is beet sugar and cane sugar, sugar from corn should be called 'corn sugar' in order to give it a name that is easily understood.

It is expected to take up to two years for the FDA to come to a decision on whether to approve the renaming. The American Dietetic Association has also found that HFCS is "nutritionally equivalent to sucrose," and that it is metabolized by the body in the same way as sucrose." [The quoted is taken from http://home. ezezene.com from *The Bee Culture*.]

[17] There is no accurate way of knowing exactly how much HFCS is actually consumed by the average American. Estimates are based on what is called the "disappearance rate," an indicator of how much of a given product "disappears" from the inventory of producers or grocery shelves. The disappearance rate is not technically the same as consumption, but it is a good estimate for one can safely assume that a food product produced for human consumption is not added to dog food or dumped down the drain.

[18] Recommended guidelines for sugars added to food products issued by the American Heart Association in March 2010.

Chapter 3

[19] Throughout this book the condensation of carbohydrates into "carbs" is used.

[20] ATP stands for adenosine-5'-trophosphate. It is often called the "molecular unit of currency" or the substance responsible for the intracellular transfer of energy. In other words, ATP transports chemical energy

within the cells as needed for cellular metabolism. [JR Knowles, "Enzyme-catalyzed phosphoryl transfer reactions," *Annual Review of Biochemistry*, (1980) **49**: 877–919]

²¹ The use of this analogy described as a "parallel reservoir management" system is credited to Mike McInnes, MRPS.

²² DJ Jenkins, TM Wolever, RH Taylor, H Barker, H Fielden, JM Baldwin, AC Bowling, HC Newman, AL Jenkins, DV Goff, "Glycemic index of foods: a physiological basis for carbohydrate exchange." *Am J Clin Nutr* (1981) 34: 362–366 (1981)

²³ PE Cryer, SN Davis, H Shamoon, "Hypoglycemia in Diabetes," *Diabetes Care* 2003 June; 26(6):1902-12

²⁴ D Jalal, MD, *et al*, "Increased fructose associates with elevated blood pressure," 2010 Sep; 21(9): 1543-9

²⁵ "Big Gulp" is a registered trademark of the 7-Eleven Company and refers to soft drinks sold in quantities from 20 to 64 ounces and larger.

Chapter 4

²⁶ *Ibid*, DJ Jenkins, *et al*

²⁷ JC Brand-Miller, K Foster-Powell, SHA Holt, "International table of glycemic index and glycemic load values: 2002," *Am J Clin Nutr* 2002; 76: 5–56

²⁸ The South Beach Diet® and the Nutrisystem® diet plans are examples of diet plans that incorporate the

GI into their recommendations. Another such diet plan called "The Low GI Revolution" was published in 2005. [J Brand-Miller, K Foster-Powell, J McMillan-Price, *"The Low GI Diet Revolution: The Defining Science-Based Weight Loss Plan."* New York; Marlow and Company, 2005

[29] Dietary Guidelines for Americans (2005), U.S. Department of Health and Agriculture. www. healthierus.gov/dietaryguidelines

[30] The glycemic index of a food is defined as the area under the two-hour blood glucose response curve (AUC) following the ingestion of a fixed portion of carbohydrate (usually 50 g). The AUC of the test food is divided by the AUC of the standard (either glucose or white bread, giving two different definitions) and then multiplied by 100. The average GI value is calculated from data collected in 10 human subjects. Both the standard and test food must contain an equal amount of available carbohydrate.

The result gives a relative ranking for each tested food. The glycemic index is a numerical index that ranks carbohydrates based on their rate of glycemic response (i.e. their rate of conversion to glucose within the human body). The glycemic index uses a scale of 0 to 100, with higher values given to foods that cause the most rapid rise in blood sugar. Pure glucose serves as a reference point, and is given a Glycemic Index (GI) of 100.

[31] http://nutritiondata.self.com/topics/glycemic-index

[32] KA Beals, PhD, "The Glycemic Index: Research Meets Reality," special publication of the United States Potato Board, October 2005

[33] *Ibid*

[34] TMS Wolever, et al, "Determination of the glycaemic index of foods: Interlaboratory study." *Eur J Clin Nutr* 2003; 57: 475-482

[35] FX Pi-Sunyer, "Glycemic index and disease," *Am J Clin Nutr* 2002; 76 (suppl): 290S-298S

[36] A Raben, et al,. Acetylation of or beta-cyclodextrin addition to potato starch: beneficial effect on glucose metabolism and appetite sensations." *Am J Clin Nutr* 1997; 66: 304-314

[37] *Ibid.*, Pi-Sunyer

[38] G Fernandes, A Velangi, TMS Wolever, "Glycemic index of potatoes commonly consumed in North America," *J Am Diet Assoc* 2005; 105: 557-562

[39] TMS Wolever, L Katzman-Relle, AL Jenkins, V Vuksan, RG Josse, DJA Jenkins, "Glycaemic index of 102 complex carbohydrate foods in patients with diabetes," *Nutr Res* 1994; 14:651-669

[40] *Ibid,* Wolever, *et al.*

[41] TMS Wolever, FQ Nuttal, R Lee, *et al*, "Prediction of the relative blood glucose response of mixed meals using the white bread glycemic index," *Diabetes Care* 1985; 8:418-428

⁴² TMS Wolever, C Bolognesi, "Time of day influences relative glycaemic effect of foods." *Nutr Res* 1996; 16: 381-384

⁴³ This section contains information summarized from the Nutrition Data website @ http://nutritiondata. self.com/topics/glycemic-index

⁴⁴ Estimated Glycemic Load or eGL™ is a registered trademark of the Nutrition Data company, NutritionData.com, 1166 Sixth Avenue, New York, NY 10036 USA

⁴⁵ Quoted from NutritionData.com Estimated Glycemic Load page

⁴⁶ *Ibid*

⁴⁷ The HPA axis or hypothalamus-pituitary-adrenal axis is a term that refers to the complex set of interactions and hormonal feedback signals between the hypothalamus – a small portion of the brain that synthesizes and secretes vasopressin and corticotropin-releasing hormone (CRH), the pituitary gland which secretes adrenocorticotropic hormone (ACTH), and the adrenal gland, which produces glucocorticoid hormones (mainly cortisol). The interactions between these organs and glands comprise the major part of the neuroendocrine system in the body that controls and regulates stress, digestion, immune system functions, emotions, sexuality, energy storage and utilization.

Chapter 5

[48] IGFBP-1 is part of what is known as the IGF Axis that includes several insulin-like growth factors (IGF), two cell-surface receptors, two bonding molecules and a family of six IGF-binding proteins along with their associated IGFBP degrading enzymes. The IGF binding proteins are known as IGFBP-1 through IGFBP-6. The IGF proteins are a series of growth and recovery factors with powerful pro-insulin activity. Their role is to rapidly drive glucose into muscle tissue. This response is emerging as a critical alarm signal warning the brain of an impending metabolic catastrophe.

When and if liver glycogen is low, IGFBP-1 is increased and inhibits IGF-1 (binds IGF-1), resulting in less glucose uptake by contracting muscles. Glucose is kept in the circulation thereby maintaining blood glucose concentration and protecting liver glycogen levels.

In a sense, IGFBP-1 is a classic stress factor released during periods when glucose supply is at a premium. In addition to this, IGFBP-1 functions as a clever metabolic signal to warn the brain of impending fuel shortage. Its release is associated with release of other stress hormones, glucagon, adrenaline and cortisol. Chronic release of IGFBP-1 is now emerging as a marker for Type 2 diabetes, which is not surprising insofar as cortisol is the other hormone most often associated with insulin resistance. IGFBP-1 levels also rise during the night fast. IGFBP-1 has also has been shown to be elevated during space flight, a form of physiologic stress associated with chronic increased metabolic stress.

[49] When bound to IGF-1, IGFBP-1 inhibits the influence of IGF-1 on human growth hormone (GH). Thus,

almost every cell in the body is affected by IGF-1, especially cells in muscle, cartilage, bone, kidney, liver, nerves, skin, and lungs. IGF-1 exerts insulin-like effects that allow for glucose (energy) to enter the cells. It also serves to regulate cell growth and development, especially in nerve cells, as well as regulating DNA synthesis in the cells.

When IGF-1 is inhibited, cellular death, rather than cell restoration and recovery, progresses unabated.

[50] "Regulation of Insulin-Like Growth Factor binding Protein-1 during the 24-Hour Metabolic clock and in Response to Hypoinsulinaemia Induced by Fasting and Sandostatin in Normal Women," *Journal of the Society for Gynecologic Investigation,* 1995

[51] In 2002, Jean-Marc Lavois established (in a study of rats during exercise) that the progressive fall in liver glycogen is indexed by increased release of IGFBP-1 into the blood circulation. This was the signal for the brain to activate the HPA axis in order to counteract the drop in glucose available for cerebral energy. This is the exercise equivalent of nocturnal diabetes in its fullest expression, where nocturnal stress will be activated as a regulatory mechanism to ensure energy for the brain.

[52] The term "liver blindness" is credited to Mike McInnes, MRPS.

Chapter 6

[53] A Peters, U Schweiger, L Pellerin, *et al,* "The selfish brain: competition for energy resources." *Neurosci Biobehav Rev* (April 2004) 28 (2): 143–80

[54] This information has been previously discussed in detail by the authors in two other books: *The Hibernation Diet*, Mike and Stuart McInnes, WorldClassEmprise, LLC (2007) and *The Honey Revolution – Restoring the Health of Future Generations*, Ron Fessenden, MD, MPH, and Mike McInnes, MRPS, WorldClassEmprise, LLC (2008).

[55] The amount of liver glycogen formed from ingesting honey is a best estimate based on the known amounts of fructose and glucose contained in honey and the relatively small elevation in blood sugar that occurs after consuming honey. The other small amounts of sugars contained in honey are not included in this estimate. These sugars would no doubt contribute to a slight but delayed rise in blood sugar as they are metabolized and absorbed into the blood farther down in the gastrointestinal tract.

[56] Note to diabetics who routinely check blood sugar in the morning on arising: don't let an elevated reading fool you. This is known as the "dawn phenomenon." Your liver glycogen reserve will be low in spite of what your blood sugar level tells you. The elevated levels of IGFBP-1 mentioned above will have alerted the brain to its impending fuel shortage. The release of cortisol from the adrenal glands would have begun the process of breaking down protein from muscle tissue into amino acids that are returned to the liver to produce new glucose. This new glucose is released into the blood and results in an artificially elevated blood sugar level in spite of the fact that your liver glycogen reserve is depleted.

Chapter 7

[57] R Fessenden, MD, MPH and M McInnes, *Smart Sleep: How to Sleep Your Way to Better Health (with Honey)*, Unpublished work (2012)

[58] Matthew 23: 24 New International Version

Chapter 8

[59] Many references for the association of metabolic stress with the conditions listed can be found in other books by the authors: *The Honey Revolution - Restoring the Health of Future Generations* and *The Honey Revolution - Abridged*, WorldClassEmprise, LLC

Elizabeth's Story

[60] For nearly 50 years, the nutritional status of the average American diet has been shifting toward a greater percentage of carbohydrates and simple sugars (some estimate that up to 80% of our total caloric intake is made up of carbohydrates and simple sugars). Ideally, our intake should contain no more than 35 to 40 percent carbohydrates, with the rest split between proteins and fats. The sad irony is that the low fat craze that drives much of our nutritional choices actually increases the risk of disease by boosting the percentage of calories that we gain from sugars.

Chapter 9

[61] Webster's Dictionary

[62] Corn is composed of more than 70% starch (or glucose), a small amount of fructose (less than a gram per cup), some sucrose (about 3 grams per cup), less than a gram per cup of other sugars, and only 5 grams of protein per cup.

[63] The reader is again referred to *The Honey Revolution – Restoring the Health of Future Generations*, by Ron Fessenden, MD, MPH and Mike McInnes, MRPS, WorldClassEmprise, LLC, 2008, for more of the facts about the disastrous results of the low-fat dietary emphasis of the past 30 years and the excessive consumption of HFCS.

[64] The HYMN cycle refers to a term used by Mike McInnes in his presentation to the First International Symposium on Honey and Health held in Sacramento, CA in 2008. The acronym refers to the HoneY-MelatoniN Cycle described on a scientific poster presented at the Symposium and reprinted in *The Honey Revolution – Restoring the Health of Future Generations*, WorldClassEmprise, LLC, 2008.

Chapter 11 – Appetizers and Snacks

[65] Adapted from "Watermelon and Blueberry Salad" by Marcella Richman, *The Buzz on Honey*, Three Bears Honey Co, Jumbo Jack's Cookbooks, August 2012.

Chapter 12 – Beverages

[66] Recipe provided by Carolyn Hock

Chapter 13 – From Salads to Salsas

[67] Adapted from *Old Favorite Honey Recipes*, American Honey Institute, Madison, Wisconsin, p.35, 1941 (Original Price - $0.10) (Book belonging to her Grandmother was donated by Carol Case, Waimeia, Hawaii)

[68] *Ibid.*, p. 36

[69] *Ibid.*, p. 10

Glenn's Story – A Happy Ending

[70] J Traynor, *Honey, The Gourmet Medicine*, Kovak Books, 2002

Appendix C

[71] *Ibid*, JC Brand-Miller, *et al* (endnote #27)

About the Author

Ron Fessenden, MD, MPH, is a retired medical doctor. He received his MD degree from the University of Kansas School of Medicine in 1970 and his Masters in Public Health from the University of Hawaii School of Public Health – Manoa in 1982.

For the past five years, Dr. Fessenden has been researching and writing about the health benefits of consuming natural honey. He has spoken at numerous venues across the United States and Canada relating to this topic, including a presentation entitled "Living Healthier – Aging Well with Honey" delivered at the Excellence in Aging Care Symposium in Fredericton, New Brunswick in September 2012.

His previous published works include:

- *The Honey Revolution — Restoring the Health of Future Generations*, WorldClassEmprise, LLC (2008) by Ron Fessenden, MD, MPH and Mike McInnes, MRPS

- *The Honey Revolution — Abridged*, WorldClassEmprise, LLC (2010) by Ron Fessenden, MD, MPH and Mike McInnes, MRPS

For more information go to:

www.tgbtgbooks.com

Or email Dr. Fessenden at:

ron@tgbtgbooks.com

CPSIA information can be obtained at www.ICGtesting.com
Printed in the USA
BVOW08s2329260713

326942BV00003BB/4/P